MW00974232

In 15 Minutes You...

Power walk (Chapter 9)
Climb stairs (Chapter 9)
Jump rope (Chapter 9)
Circuit train (Chapter 9)
Strength train with resistance bands (Chapter 10)

- ➤ Leg press
- ➤ Seated row
- ➤ Chest press
- ➤ Lateral raise

- ➤ Biceps curl
- ➤ Triceps extension
- ➤ Reverse crunches
- ➤ Crunches

In 30 Minutes You Can:

Interval train (Chapter 11)
Do a mini-triathlon (Chapter 11)
Strength train (Chapter 12)

- ➤ Leg press
- ➤ Leg curl
- ➤ Leg extension
- ➤ Lat pulldown
- ➤ Upright rows
- ➤ Chest press
- ➤ Dips

- ➤ Shoulder press
- ➤ Seated biceps curl
- ➤ Triceps push down
- ➤ Reverse crunch
- ➤ Crunch
- ➤ Back raise

In 45 Minutes You Can:

Do a full workout (Chapter 13):

- ➤ Warm up (5 minutes)
- ➤ Cardio (15 minutes)
- ➤ Cool down (5 minutes)

- ➤ Strength train (15 minutes)
- ➤ Stretch (5 minutes)

Do a full cardio workout (Chapter 14)
Do a full strength training workout (Chapter 15)
Add these exercises to the 30-minute workout:

- ➤ Standing calf raise
- ➤ Flyes

- ➤ Lateral raises
- ➤ Oblique crunches

tear here

alpha books

In 60 Minutes You Can:

Do a full workout (Chapter 16):
- ➤ Warm up (5 minutes)
- ➤ Cardio (20 minutes)
- ➤ Cool down (5 minutes)
- ➤ Strength train (25 minutes)
- ➤ Stretch (5 minutes)

Take an exercise class (Chapter 17)
Do a full cardio workout (Chapter 17)
Do a full strength training routine (Chapter 18)
Add these exercises to the 45-minute workout:
- ➤ Add seated calf raise
- ➤ Dips
- ➤ Concentration curls
- ➤ Triceps kickback

Do a split routine (Chapter 18)

Workout Tips

Don't bounce when you stretch.

Don't stretch to the point of pain.

Hold your stretches for 20 to 30 seconds.

Lift using slow, controlled movements.

Don't hold your breath when lifting.

Use a spotter when necessary.

Stay within your heart rate training zone during cardio workouts.

Never skip your warm up or cool down.

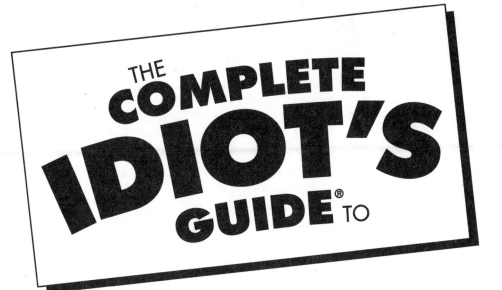

THE COMPLETE IDIOT'S GUIDE® TO

Short Workouts

by Deidre Johnson-Cane, Jonathan Cane,
and Joe Glickman

alpha books

Macmillan USA, Inc.
201 West 103rd Street
Indianapolis, IN 46290

A Pearson Education Company

To our families, our friends, and our readers.

Copyright © 2001 by Deidre Johnson-Cane, Jonathan Cane, and Joe Glickman

International Standard Book Number: 0-02-863953-7
Library of Congress Catalog Card Number: Available upon request.

03   02   01   8   7   6   5   4   3

Interpretation of the printing code: The rightmost number of the first series of numbers is the year of the book's printing; the rightmost number of the second series of numbers is the number of the book's printing. For example, a printing code of 01-1 shows that the first printing occurred in 2001.

Printed in the United States of America

Publisher
Marie Butler-Knight

Product Manager
Phil Kitchel

Managing Editor
Cari Luna

Senior Acquisitions Editor
Renee Wilmeth

Development Editor
Joan D. Paterson

Production Editor
Billy Fields

Copy Editor
Faren Bachelis

Illustrator
Jody P. Schaeffer

Cover Designers
Mike Freeland
Kevin Spear

Book Designers
Scott Cook and Amy Adams of DesignLab

Photographer
Peter Baiamonte

Indexer
Lisa Wilson

Layout/Proofreading
Angela Calvert
Svetlana Dominguez
Lizbeth Patterson

Contents at a Glance

Part 1: The Basics   **1**

1   Why Try Short Workouts?   3
Getting in shape in far less time than you think.

2   Fitting It In   13
Finding the time to work out.

3   Workouts and Your Body   27
How your body responds to different types of exercise.

4   Nutrition   41
Eating right on the go.

Part 2: The Components of Fitness   **53**

5   Aerobics   55
Sweating it out for cardiovascular health.

6   Strengthening   65
The basics of muscle building.

7   Start with Stretching   75
Staying limber and loose.

8   Working Out with Babies and Toddlers   89
Parenthood doesn't mean the end of your health.

Part 3: The Workouts: 15 Minutes to 30 Minutes   **101**

9   The 15-Minute Cardio Workout   103
Burning calories in just 15 minutes.

10   The 15-Minute Strength-Training Workout   111
Quick muscle-building workouts.

11   The 30-Minute Cardio Workout   125
Half-hour workouts for your heart and lungs.

12   The 30-Minute Strength-Training Workout   133
Muscle-building strategies in 30 minutes.

Part 4: The Workouts: 45 Minutes to 60 Minutes   **149**

13   The 45-Minute Workout   151
Putting it all together in 45 minutes.

14   The 45-Minute Cardio Workout   159
Forty-five minutes of calorie burning.

15 The 45-Minute Strength-Training Workout   167
    Thorough weight-training routines.

16 The 60-Minute Workout   189
    Full workouts you can do in an hour.

17 The 60-Minute Cardio Workout   197
    Hour-long aerobic regimes.

18 The Hour of Power   207
    Full one-hour strengthening plans.

19 Don't Waste Your Time   221
    Avoiding the most common pitfalls in the gym.

20 Weekend Warrior—Conditioning for Sports   235
    Sports-specific exercise routines.

Part 5: Away from the Gym   249

21 Working Out on the Road   251
    Exercise strategies when you're away from home.

22 Five-Minute Workouts at the Office   261
    What to do when you're stuck at your desk.

23 The Workout Wardrobe   275
    Stylish and effective clothing and equipment options.

24 Seasonal Workouts   287
    Exercising in hot or cold conditions.

Appendixes

A Glossary   297

B Resource Guide   301

   Index   305

Contents

Part 1: The Basics   **1**

1 Why Try Short Workouts?   **3**

Pick Up the Pace 4
Something vs. Nothing 5
   Belief Number 1. False. 6
   Belief Number 2. False, Falser, and Most False. 6
   Belief Number 3. False, Unless You Know What You're Doing. 6
   Belief Number 4. False. 6
Top Ten Reasons to Work Out 7
Stress Management 7
   Hear the Hormones 8
   Work Out Your Stress 8
Keeping Up Good Habits 9
Keep It Moving 9
Head Games 10
Physically Speaking 11
How Can 15, 30, or 60 Minutes Be Enough? 11

2 Fitting It In   **13**

Excuses, Excuses 14
Time Management 14
Finding the Time 16
For Early Birds Only 18
How About Lunch? 20
After Work Workouts 20
   On the Run 21
   Work Out at Work 21
   On the Road Again 21
Setting Goals 22
   Why Develop Your Cardiovascular Fitness? 22
   Why Build Up Your Physical Strength? 23
   Why Extend Your Flexibility? 24
Values-Based Prioritizing 24

3 Workouts and Your Body   **27**

What's Up, Doc? 27
   Hypertension 29
   Diabetes 29
   Asthma 30
Measuring Your Fitness Level 31
   Resting Heart Rate 32
   Weight and Body Composition 33

Muscular Strength and Endurance 34
Cardiovascular Tests 35
Flexibility 36
Looking Good 37
Feeling Healthy 37
Being Strong 37
How Your Body Responds to Exercise 38
Cardiovascular Exercise 38
Strength Training 39
Stretching 39
Weight Loss 39
Detraining—Missing Workouts 40

4 Nutrition   **41**

Know Your Nutrients 41
General Nutrition Guidelines 43
Consuming Your Carbohydrates 44
It's the Berries 44
Eat Your Veggies 44
Protein and Its Alternatives 45
Devouring Dairy Products 45
Yum, Yum 46
Servings on the Road 46
V Is for Vitamins 51
Water, Water Everywhere 52

Part 2: The Components of Fitness   **53**

5 Aerobics   **55**

Your Cardiovascular System 55
Define Your CV Goals 56
ACSM Minimum Requirements 57
Your Target Heart Rate 58
How Long Is a Heartbeat? 59
Eating Before Workouts 60
Choosing Your CV Machine 61
Classy Exercise 62
Spin, Baby, Spin 62
Step It Up 63
Aerobics Class 63

6 Strengthening   **65**

The Strength Debate 66
Muscle Turns Heads 66
Faster Metabolisms Burn Calories 67
Ouch Control 67

Life 101 68
   Sad But True 68
Principled Strength 69
   Choice of Exercise 69
   Progression of Exercise 69
   Frequency 69
   Sets 70
   Reps 70
   Weight 70
   Speed of Movement 70
   Rest Between Sets 70
Working Out at Home 71
   Free Weights 73

7 Start with Stretching   **75**

Why Me? 76
Stretching 101 77
Sidestep Injury 77
The Basic Stretches 78
   Quadriceps 78
   Hamstrings 79
   Lower and Middle Back Muscles 80
   Hip Flexors 83
   Groin 84
   Calves 85
   Pectorals 86
Where Does Yoga Fit In? 87

8 Working Out with Babies and Toddlers   **89**

Oh, Momma! 90
The Big Comeback 91
Start Me Up 92
   Strengthening the Pelvic Wall 92
   Audacious Abdominals 92
   Tighten Those Gluteals 93
Joining a Postpartum Class 93
Baby, Let's Stroll 93
Two for One 94
Cardio Partner Time 94
Strength Training with Your Partner 94
Working Out with Baby 95
   Rocking Out with Your Baby 95
   A Bicycle Built for Mom and Baby 95
   Baby Bicycle Seats 96
   Baby Trailers 97
   Jog, Baby 98

Part 3: The Workouts: 15 Minutes to 30 Minutes   101

9 The 15-Minute Cardio Workout   103

Left Foot, Right Foot 103
Jump Rope: Not Just for Kids and Boxers 104
  Choosing a Rope 105
  Types of Rope 105
Upstairs, Downstairs 107
Short Circuit 108

10 The 15-Minute Strength-Training Workout   111

Band on the Run 111
Crunch Time 115
Reverse Crunches 116
A Helping Hand 116
Remember Calisthenics? 120
  Proper Push-Ups 121
  Chin-Ups and Pull-Ups 121
  Learn to Lunge 122
Creative Calisthenics 123

11 The 30-Minute Cardio Workout   125

Incorporate Intervals into Your Workout 126
Running Workouts 126
  Progress from Power Walking to Running 128
Ride Workouts 128
  Stand and Deliver 129
  Turn on the Spin Cycle 129
Tri This 130
  Indoor or Out 130
  Think Vertical 131

12 The 30-Minute Strength-Training Workout   133

Upper-Body Emphasis 133
  Leg Press 134
  Lat Pull Down 135
  Upright Row 137
  Chest/Bench Press 138
  Dips 139
  Shoulder Press 141
  Seated Biceps Curl 142
  Triceps Push Down 143
  Back Raise 144
Lower-Body Emphasis 145
  Leg Curl 145
  Leg Extension 147

Part 4: The Workouts: 45 Minutes to 60 Minutes   149

13   The 45-Minute Workout   151

The Breakdown 152
Get Warm 152
Cardiovascular Workouts 154
Cooldown 155
Stretching 156
Strength Training 157

14   The 45-Minute Cardio Workout   159

Fun Running 159
Ride Like the Wind 162
Go Row 162
No-Impact Workouts 163
  Elliptical Trainers *163*
  Ski Cross-Country Indoors *164*

15   The 45-Minute Strength-Training Workout   167

Upper-Body Emphasis 167
  Flyes *168*
  Lateral Raises *170*
  Oblique Crunch *171*
Lower-Body Emphasis 172
  Squat *173*
  Abduction *175*
  Adduction *176*
  Standing Calf Raise *177*
Split Personality 178
Days One and Four 178
  Incline Press *179*
  Decline Press *180*
  Triceps Kickback *182*
Days Two and Five 183
  Dumbbell Rows *183*
  Shrugs *185*
  Concentration Curls *186*

16   The 60-Minute Workout   189

It's About Time 190
The Workout 190
  Going Up? *190*
  Sitting Down on the Job *191*
Lifting 193
Stretching the Truth 194

17 The 60-Minute Cardio Workout   **197**

Run for Your Life 198
Training for a Marathon 198
Time for a Ride 201
Training for a Century Ride 202
Show Some Class 204
Spin Your Wheels 204
Step to the Beat 205
Have Fun 206

18 The Hour of Power   **207**

The All-in-One Hour 208
Seated Calf Raise 208
Which Way to the Beach? 209
Nice Legs 211
Split Personality 212
Push/Pull Split Routine 212
Standing Biceps Curl 213
Front Raises 215
Reverse Flyes 216
French Curls 217

19 Don't Waste Your Time   **221**

Cardio No-No's 222
Cheating on the StairMaster 222
Holding On for Dear Life 222
Hang Loose 223
Standing Toe Touch 223
Hurdler's Stretch 224
Yoga Plough 225
Strength 225
Bad Crunch Form 225
Good Crunch Form 226
Exploding Myths 227
Double Leg Lift with Straight Legs 227
Bad Bench Press Form 228
Some More No-No's 229
Barbell Bent Rows, Good Mornings, and
  Stiff-Legged Dead Lifts 230
A Zillion Leg Lifts 231
Full Sit-Ups 231
Arching Back for Biceps Curls 232

20 Weekend Warrior—Conditioning for Sports   235

Running 236
Cycling 238
Tennis 239
Golf 241
Skating 242
Skiing/Snowboarding 244
Martial Arts 245
Paddling 246

Part 5:   Away from the Gym   249

21 Working Out on the Road   251

Seek and Ye Shall Find 252
Gym-less in Seattle 252
Cals *253*
Jumping Rope *253*
Push-Ups *253*
Pull-Ups and Chin-Ups *254*
Resistance Bands *254*
Overcoming Jet Lag 254
High Altitude 257
Working Out in Bad Weather 258

22 Five-Minute Workouts at the Office   261

Carpal Tunnel Syndrome 262
Perfect Posture 263
Take a Seat *264*
Proper Workstation Posture *265*
Setting Up an Ergonomically Efficient Workstation *265*
Combating Neck, Back, and Shoulder Pain 266
Stretching at Your Desk 267
Strengthening at Your Desk 270
Stair Workouts 271
Calisthenics Are Convenient 272
Performing Push-Ups *272*
Contract/Relax Technique 273

23 The Workout Wardrobe   275

Threads 275
Form Meets Content 276
Running Shorts *276*
Cycling Shorts *276*
For Women Only: Sports Bras *277*

Singlets 277
Socks 277
Material Matters 277
Lycra/Spandex 278
Cotton 278
CoolMax 278
Lively in Layers 279
Base Layer 279
Insulating Layer 280
Outer Layer 280
Dress Code 280
At Home 280
At the Gym 280
On the Road 281
Shoes 281
Fitting Your Foot 282
Match Your Shoe to What You Do 282
Don't Resist Resistance Bands 283
Ankle Weights Are Awesome 284

24 Seasonal Workouts   287

Stay Warm in the Cold 288
Winter Wonders 289
Ice-Skating 289
Skiing 290
Cross-Country Skiing 290
Snowboarding 290
Staying Cool When It's Hot 290
Heat Cramps 291
Heat Exhaustion 291
Heatstroke 292
Summer Sweatin' 292
Swimming 292
Running 293
In-Line Skating 294
Cycling 294
Mountain Bikes 294
Road Bikes 295
Hybrids 295

Appendixes

A Glossary   297

B Resource Guide   301

Index   305

Foreword

Unlike some folks I know —and unlike some of my best running partners over the years—I've never been one of those people who needs to be prodded to work out. While I've always loved exercising, like so many others, I'm faced with the constant challenge of balancing my professional obligations, my family life, and my fitness. Today, at age 45, as a married man with three children and a busy work schedule, I no longer have the time to work out for hours on end. Still, with a little creativity and planning, I'm able to find ways to work out on a consistent basis and remain a competitive athlete.

My exercise methods might not be conventional, but I've found that they work for me. While my travel schedule might seem like a deterrent to exercising, I've found that the best way to get a sense of a city is with a vigorous run through town. You discover stuff no tourist sees.

My wife and I have begun the regular practice of stretching together for 15 minutes at night. It allows us to spend some quality time together and helps us stay injury free.

I've even found myself at the local high school track doing what I call "kid intervals"—running laps with my two oldest children. During my harder efforts, they play on the infield, and during my recovery laps they run the track with me.

In *The Complete Idiot's Guide to Short Workouts,* you'll find a variety of practical time-saving tips that can help you incorporate exercise into your busy lifestyle. In fact, while the book is full of sound guidance and scientific exercise principles as well as photos to clearly demonstrate proper form, what sets it apart from so many other fitness publications is that the authors recognize that most people can't dedicate all day to working out. This *Guide* provides you with ideas for everything from quick stretches you can do at your desk to strategies for exercising while you're on the road. It even has tips for training for a marathon or century bicycle ride with limited gym time.

By following the guidelines presented in *The Complete Idiot's Guide to Short Workouts,* you'll learn what I've found out through experience—staying in shape (or getting in shape) isn't just for childless lottery winners with fully equipped gyms in their basement. It's possible to balance your professional obligations, family life, and a fitness routine and still get some sleep at night. That balancing act is made much easier with the guidance you'll find here.

—Tom Phillips

Tom Phillips is CEO of Deja.com and has served as president of ESPN and ABC News Internet divisions. In 1985, he co-founded *Spy* magazine. At age 45, Mr. Phillips is a competitive runner and fitness enthusiast and the father of three children aged 9, 6, and 3.

Introduction

Way back in the twentieth century, the main problem faced by those of us who tried to encourage people to exercise was convincing them of the many benefits of working out. Whether it was the talk of decreased injury, lower blood pressure, or just plain good looks, by the time the century came to a close, millions of Americans were believers. Unfortunately, many of these converts found themselves faced with a new set of challenges: balancing 60-hour work weeks, family life, and an attempt at a social life left precious little time to exercise.

We've all seen the hyperbole-filled TV infomercials that stop just short of promising to transform a couch potato into a pro beach volleyball player with just eight minutes of exercise a day. We've also seen the movie-star action hero who works out four hours a day to achieve that implausibly gorgeous body. Luckily for us real people, there's something in-between. That's where we come in.

While we're not so bold as to claim that the short workouts that we outline will perform miracles, we're confident that they can help you toward your fitness goals. As you read this book, you'll find everything from quick exercises you can do at your desk or in your hotel room to thorough 60-minute gym routines. Maybe 15 minutes of jumping rope and stretching isn't as good as a two-hour session at a state-of-the-art gym, but it sure beats wolfing a doughnut while you sit at your computer monitor wishing you had more time to exercise.

How This Book Is Organized

The Complete Idiot's Guide to Short Workouts is organized into five parts. We start with fitness basics and your needs and then lead you into the cardiovascular, strength, and flexibility routines that you can perform in a limited time.

Part 1, "The Basics," takes a look at the value of short workouts and how to fit a workout—even as short as 15 minutes—into your busy day. Chapter 2 gets you started by explaining the physical and psychological value of even very short periods of exercise. In Chapter 2, you'll discover fragments of time that you can put to good use with a short workout. Chapter 3 assesses your needs and helps you measure your fitness level and define your goals. We'll give you the lowdown on how your body responds to different types of exercise as well as what happens when you miss workouts. Then, in Chapter 4, we'll discuss your eating habits and review healthful nutrition recommendations.

Part 2, "The Components of Fitness," describes the major components of fitness: cardiovascular endurance, strength, and flexibility. Chapter 5 explains how to calculate your target heart rate and reviews different kinds of aerobic classes. Chapter 6 gives some solid reasons for taking strength training seriously, and Chapter 7 reviews some basic but oh-so-important stretches. In Chapter 8, parents of youngsters will find strategies for combining child care and fitness.

Part 3, "The Workouts: 15 Minutes to 30 Minutes," gives you ideas on how to break a sweat in 15 minutes. In Chapter 9, you'll realize that walking, jumping rope, and climbing stairs can increase your cardiovascular fitness as well as a 15-minute circuit-training workout. Chapter 10 discusses resistance bands, working with a partner, and good old calisthenics to give you 15 minutes of strength training. In Chapter 11 you'll learn about the benefits of interval training and find out how to do a three-minute triathlon. Chapter 12 outlines a half-hour strength-training workout, complete with photos and tips.

Part 4, "The Workouts: 45 Minutes to 60 Minutes," shows you what you can do with a little more time. Chapter 13 reveals that 45 minutes is plenty for an efficient and effective workout. Chapter 14 is dedicated to three-quarters of an hour of cardio workouts and Chapter 15 details a variety of muscle-building routines for upper and lower body that you can complete in 45 minutes. Chapter 16 outlines a full hour of cardio, strength, and flexibility routines. Chapters 17 and 18 describe what you can achieve with an hour dedicated to cardio training and muscle building, respectively. Chapter 19 explains how to exercise correctly and which exercises to avoid. Chapter 20 will get you in condition to play your favorite weekend sports.

Part 5, "Away from the Gym," shows you how to keep exercising when you are not able to get to the gym or do your usual workout at home. Chapter 21 outlines strategies for working out when you are traveling and Chapter 22 gives five-minutes workouts you can do at the office. Chapter 23 looks at what to wear for comfort and ease while working out and Chapter 24 provides information on how to safely exercise under changing weather conditions.

Extras

Additional information is presented alongside the text. You'll find sidebars in each chapter containing four types of informational inserts.

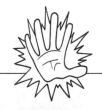

Stop Short

This sidebar highlights issues that ensure that you have a safe workout. Heeding these warnings will help you stay free of pain and injury.

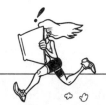

Info to Go

These sidebars contain tidbits and anecdotes that you might find fun and informative.

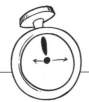

Short Cuts

Tips to make your exercise a little more effective and efficient. These pointers alert you to little things that can make the difference between a so-so workout and a great one.

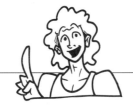

Workout Words

Here you'll find clear, concise definitions of new terms introduced in the text. You may have a hard time working your new vocabulary into dinner conversation, but it will help in the gym.

Acknowledgments

Putting a book together can test friendships and weaken one's grip on sanity. Thankfully (especially for the married couples among us), we've managed to do it again. With-out the invaluable help of some great colleagues and friends, it would have been impossible. Among them are our models: Barrie Lifton, Lauralee Giovanella, Sejal Vyas, Aristides Maisonave, David Duhan, and Chris Zogopolous. You're good-looking and work cheap—what could be better? Thanks also go out to Susanne Elstein, a talented and forgiving photographer. Special thanks to Ralph Anastasio of New York's Printing House Fitness Center for his continued support.

Deidre thanks her father, Robert, and her sister, Lynette, for their love and support.

Special thanks from Jonathan to his family, his coauthors, and all his teachers, with-out whom he'd never have the nerve to try half of the things he does.

Joe wishes to thank his wife, Beth, and beautiful daughter, Willa, who, at age four, will soon be correcting her Dad's spelling.

Trademarks

All terms mentioned in this book that are known to be or are suspected of being trademarks or service marks have been appropriately capitalized. Alpha Books and Macmillan USA, Inc., cannot attest to the accuracy of this information. Use of a term in this book should not be regarded as affecting the validity of any trademark or service mark.

Part 1

The Basics

In this part, we'll do our best to convince you that you can be healthy and fit without giving up your job, disowning your family, or having your mail sent to the gym. No matter how jam-packed your work and social calendar may be, we'll help you get and stay fit in far less time than you may have thought possible.

Short workouts can be effective in helping you gain and maintain fitness, and some exercise is almost always better than none. Once we've made our compelling case for short workouts, we'll help you fit them into your busy schedule. We'll give you the lowdown on how your body responds to different types of exercise as well as what happens when you miss workouts. We'll provide guidelines for healthful nutrition and tips on how to eat out without blowing your diet.

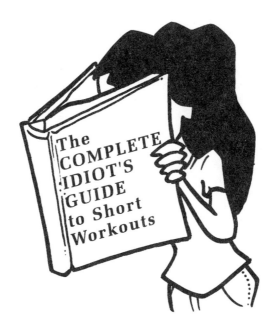

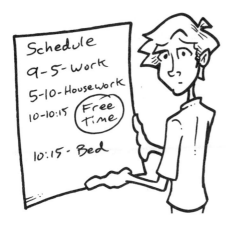

Chapter 1

Why Try Short Workouts?

In This Chapter

➤ Efficient workouts save time

➤ Short workouts are better than no workouts

➤ Exercise is the best stress-buster

➤ Exercise keeps you going

While we assume there are a few people out there who would rather be built like Bugs Bunny instead of Michael Jordan or, say, Olive Oyl rather than Jessica Rabbit, most of us would take svelte over soft, firm over flabby. The issue for most of us isn't desire. Few people who have ever worked out doubt that exercise is good for your body and mind. The problem for most of us over the age of 21 isn't why or how to work out, but when. Ironically, when you were young and had ample time to work out, you didn't really need to.

Without a doubt, the most common reason people offer as to why they miss workouts (or give up exercise entirely) is the ubiquitous "I'm too busy" refrain. While this is a legitimate excuse—the time constraints of work and family are considerable—with regard to health, it's the biggest mistake one can make.

Lean-and-mean screen stars such as Sly Stallone, Arnold Schwarzenegger, Linda Hamilton, and Jamie Lee Curtis can work out all day like mules plowing a dry field—and why not, their bodies are their meal tickets. But the bottom line is that you can maintain, and even improve, your fitness on less than one hour a day.

Pick Up the Pace

The cowriters of this book admit they're workout fanatics. Among their friends, the husband-and-wife team of Jonathan and Deidre are known as Mr. and Ms. Endorphin. Deidre is a former two-time national and world power-lifting champ who makes her living as a physical therapist. Jonathan is a competitive cyclist, multisport enthusiast, and exercise physiologist who actually looks forward to footraces up the Empire State Building.

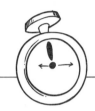

Short Cuts

A good way to keep track of time in the gym is to get a digital watch. Start the timer as you enter the gym and pay close attention to your rest periods.

The most frequently asked question they get is "What is the most common mistake people make in the gym?" Much to nearly everyone's surprise, their answer is "People spend too much time in the gym!" It's an answer that often elicits an eloquent wide-eyed response: "Huh?"

The reason so many people are taken by surprise is that more often than not even busy gym rats spend too much time schmoozing and not enough time taking care of their fitness business. (Don't get us wrong: Gyms are great places to socialize. In fact, Jonathan and Deidre met over the leg extension machine at the Hunter College Gym in Manhattan, but Jonathan insists that he never stopped doing leg extensions while they chatted.)

In the pages that follow we'll show you how you can build a physique you'll be proud of without spending half your free time in the gym. We also educate you on how you can improve your cardiovascular fitness without logging major treadmill hours.

Don't get the wrong idea. Working out an hour a day won't have you auditioning as Wesley Snipes's body double in his next film or as Xena in her next TV adventure. Nor are you likely to qualify for the Boston Marathon on a handful of cardio hours a week. To compete with the big boys and girls requires a significant investment in time and effort. When Deidre competed as a power lifter, she logged one to four hours a day pumping iron, stretching, and doing cardio workouts. Joe Glickman, the third wheel in our writing team and a two-time member of the U.S. National Marathon Team, routinely crams his six-foot-four frame into a tippy kayak 12 to 15 hours a week when he's preparing for a big paddling marathon. (And he trains less than many of the guys on the squad.)

The moral of the story is obvious: Big results require big effort. But after years of cramming in workouts at all hours of the day, we've become masters of workout efficiency. Our aim in this book is to show you how to feel and look great as well as reduce your stress level on a far more modest allotment of that precious commodity: time.

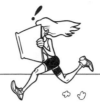

Info to Go

Perhaps one of the reasons so many people with noble workout intentions don't break a sweat on a regular basis is that their expectations are out of whack. Open any health-and-fitness magazine and you're confronted with scores of models with bulging pecs, abs of steel, and pearly whites to boot. Anyone who's spent time pumping iron knows that such physiques are hard to come by. As a result, they assume that if they don't work out three hours a day, they won't measure up to the buff bod in the underwear ads. No, an hour a day won't get you into Calvin Klein's next ad campaign, but it will make significant improvements in how you look and feel.

Something vs. Nothing

One of the key points to remember is that doing something is always better than doing nothing. Once you eliminate the mindset that you have to hammer like a galley slave for two hours or more a day, you've already cleared a significant mental hurdle. We'll help you tackle your fitness obstacles by ...

➤ Giving you sample workouts you can do in as little as 15 minutes.

➤ Fine-tuning your workouts to maximize results.

➤ Helping you manage your time and squeeze in workouts before or after work, or even on your lunch hour.

➤ Providing workouts that you can do without going to the gym.

➤ Offering a variety of stress-busting stretches that you can do at your desk.

➤ Providing you with nutritional guidelines for eating at home, in restaurants, or even on a plane.

➤ Detailing workout options you can fall back on when you hit the road on business or vacation.

Next thing you know you'll be doing short workouts three times a day and start thinking about entering a triathlon. But before we begin turning you into a maven of workout efficiency, here's an insightful quiz we'd like you to take:

True	False		
❏	❏	1.	The only way to maintain an exercise program is by going to the gym.
❏	❏	2.	The longer you spend in the gym, the more productive you are.
❏	❏	3.	Fifteen to thirty minutes of exercise a day isn't worth the bother.
❏	❏	4.	Once you become a parent, get promoted, or run for the U.S. Senate you can kiss exercise good-bye.

Here's how you should have replied:

Belief Number 1. False.

Yes, it's wonderful that we live in a culture where health clubs are nearly everywhere, but there are roughly 874 options to get and stay fit that don't involve the gym. (In fact, in prehistoric days there were very few indoor gyms and most of those old-timers were able to chase a woolly mammoth for miles.)

Belief Number 2. False, Falser, and Most False.

Often there's an inverse relationship between how long you stay and how fit you are—as in, the longer you stay the less fit you are. Check it out, next time some lean-and-mean lifting type walks into the gym, glance at the clock and see how long he stays in the gym. More often than not, he's a model of efficiency—in and out in less than an hour. More often than not, many "gym rats" work out wagging their tongues more than they do working their muscles.

Belief Number 3. False, Unless You Know What You're Doing.

Significant cardiovascular or strength benefits can be gained in 15 or 30 minutes if you know what you are doing. In fact, if you spend much more than 45 minutes lifting weights during one session you're probably wasting time.

Belief Number 4. False.

The irony here is that the busier you are, the more you need to exercise. That's because exercise reduces stress, boosts your energy, and improves your health. When you're busy you can't afford to get sick. The fact is that working out is excellent preventive medicine. Again, you're not training to climb Everest, just to get or stay in shape, which in our culture has become a rather "lofty" goal.

Top Ten Reasons to Work Out

Let's get a bit more specific about why you can't afford not to work out. Exercise …

1. Improves your appearance as well as your self-esteem.

2. Lowers your blood pressure and reduces the risk of heart disease.

3. Makes your muscles, joints, and bones stronger. This is particularly important for women over 40 who lose bone density as they age.

4. Is practical: Carrying groceries or your kids, or changing a tire are far easier when you've got some oomph.

5. Reduces stress and helps people counteract depression. For a society that pops Prozac and other psychotropic drugs like candy, that's significant.

6. Improves your ability to concentrate.

7. Increases your levels of HDL, the good *cholesterol*.

8. Improves your sleep.

9. Speeds up your metabolism—a huge factor in a country with more obese people than any other in the Western world.

10. Keeps the stock market on an even keel. Well, maybe not, but the preceding nine reasons are legit.

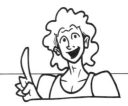

Workout Words

Cholesterol is a hormone manufactured by the liver. It is an important component of cell membranes and is necessary in repairing cell membranes and manufacturing vitamin D on the skin's surface.

Stress Management

There's been tons written on the biggest, baddest, and most silent killer in our society today: stress. Many health experts feel stress has more to do with disease than any other single factor. In our fast-paced, industrialized world we're surrounded by umpteen factors that can get our blood pressure rising: finding a job, apartment, or spouse; dealing

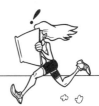

Info to Go

Not all stress is bad. In fact, often stress is necessary and helpful. Trying to, say, lose weight or learn how to rock climb may leave you temporarily anxious, but the opportunity to challenge yourself for a healthy aim is well worth it.

with hostile co-workers, traffic, tidal waves, invading armies, and more. Even "good" stress like getting married or moving into a plush new home can leave you frazzled.

There are many strategies to deal with stress (and many books that deal exhaustively with the subject), but one common problem we find with people who suffer from chronic stress is a feeling of little or no control in their life. One simple but very effective way to gain a sense of control is to plan your day so that you exercise regularly. Even if you're doing a short but brisk 30-minute workout, the sense that you're doing something "just for you" is incredibly therapeutic.

Hear the Hormones

When you're under stress, two hormones, *cortisol* and *adrenaline,* are released in your body. During extended stressful periods of time, excessive amounts of these hormones are emitted, often with rather devastating effects:

➤ Depression of cartilage and bone formation.

➤ Inhibition of the inflammatory response.

➤ Depression of the immune system.

➤ Changes in cardiovascular, neural, and gastrointestinal function.

➤ Increased blood pressure.

➤ Weight gain.

➤ Depression.

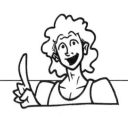

Workout Words

Cortisol, or hydrocortisol, is a hormone released by the adrenal cortex. It is closely related to cortisone in physiological effects as an anti-inflammatory agent. **Adrenaline** is known as the "fight-or-flight" hormone.

Remember the all-nighters you pulled in college or when you had to prepare for one of the most important meetings of your career? Odds are, soon after the event was over you got sick. That's because high amounts of stress-induced cortisol lowered your immune system making you more susceptible to getting sick.

What does all this have to do with exercise? Exercise can help reduce your stress, which will in turn reduce high levels of cortisol in your body.

Work Out Your Stress

We've already talked about how exercise helps you deal with stress—30 purposeful minutes of lifting or a brisk walk in the park can do wonders to soothe the savage beast. When you experience the dramatic changes in both your mood and overall state of well-being, you'll be amazed.

One often-overlooked point is the importance of finding the activity (or activities) that suit you best. If you know that running or an aerobics class is just what the doctor ordered, but you absolutely loathe running or group activities, you're actually adding to the stress level in your life. Experiment with the variety of options at your disposal: in-line skating, hiking with your dog, ultimate Frisbee, mountain or road biking, and soccer are just a few. As the philosopher Joseph Campbell said, "Follow your bliss."

Keeping Up Good Habits

Anyone who's ever started an exercise program knows it's difficult to begin and easy to stop. For most of us the demands of work, family, illness, and more threaten to derail even the best intentioned among us. The key is to stay focused on your goal of good health and fitness.

In the chapters that follow, we'll show you how you can carry on with your exercise program when you have to put your normal routine on hold. Armed with the right tools and attitude, you can seamlessly transition from your normal routine to the proverbial bump in the road and back to your routine again. In Chapters 21, "Working Out on the Road," and 22, "Five-Minute Workouts at the Office," we'll offer plenty of ideas of how to handle your workout when you hit the road or when your boss throws a folder the size of an encyclopedia on your desk on Friday at 4 o'clock and matter-of-factly asks you for a full report by Monday morning.

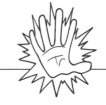

Stop Short

Too often people just starting to work out let temporary setbacks throw them off the fitness trail. Follow the model of one of the most determined athletes on the planet—a child learning to walk. Think of fitness as a lifetime activity that is built around joy and play, not work and deprivation.

Keep It Moving

Stu Mittleman, an exercise physiologist who happens to be one of the best ultradistance runners in America, typically runs 20 miles a day, six, even seven days a week. (An ultra marathon is any race over 26.2 miles.) In 1986, Mr. Mittleman set a world record by running 1,000 miles in under 12 days. When Joe was interviewing him for a profile, even he was amazed how he was able to endure so many miles on his slight frame. "Why," Joe asked, "do you run 20 miles every day?" Without pausing, Mittleman said, "Because I don't have time for more." While few of us will ever run that much in a week let alone one day, Middleman's point is sound— our bodies are made to move. Still skeptical?

This explains why being inert for hours at a time feels so bad. Just think about how you feel at after a long airline flight or when you're tied to your desk all day: Your back, neck, and shoulders hurt. The same holds true when you oversleep. Often you feel hung over. Only when you get up and go are you able to shake the cobwebs and feel more energetic.

While this sounds counterintuitive, when you're inactive for too long, your circulation becomes sluggish, your joints become stiff, and your muscles tighten up. This physical discomfort clouds your ability to concentrate on the task at hand. Confined to your seat, you start rolling your shoulders, swiveling your head, jiggling your legs—anything to try and jump-start your stalled engine. The moral of the story? Stop sitting around so much and move. And here's the obvious but oft-neglected point: Do something you enjoy.

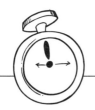

Short Cuts

Early in your workout career, the best way to motivate yourself is to think about how good you'll feel when you're done. Once exercise becomes part of your routine, your body will crave it. In other words, early on, use your mind to motivate you; later, listen to your body.

Head Games

Sports psychologists tell us that your mind is 85 percent responsible for whether you win or lose, succeed or fail. This is why it is important to prepare yourself psychologically for virtually everything you do. Integrating exercise into your life is no exception.

Psychologically, working out offers a handful of invaluable benefits.

➤ Exercising for as little as 15 minutes in a day can rev up a sluggish system by increasing circulation and oxygen intake as well as removing metabolic waste from muscles. This boost of energy comes from the release of *endorphins,* which reduces (or alleviates) stress and provides you with a feeling of well-being.

➤ Exercising for even short segments reminds you that you're involved in a healthy lifestyle. In other words, by making sure you weave physical activity into the fabric of your life you're more likely to become conscious of what you're eating and whether you're drinking enough water.

➤ Working out with others is a great way to meet positive-thinking people. In addition, hooking up with a partner or two usually means you won't miss a workout.

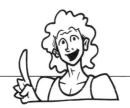

Workout Words

Endorphins are natural opiates, which become elevated in the body during exercise. They are responsible for providing you with a sense of well-being. Hence the term endorphin junkie.

Physically Speaking

Not that you needed convincing, but let's say that we've convinced you more that exercise can help you psychologically. Now let's list a few of the physical reasons why you should work out:

➤ **Exercise encourages blood flow.** Blood flow removes metabolic waste from tissues and provides fresh oxygen. When blood flow is restricted, metabolic waste builds up in the tissues and oxygen flow is restricted. Want to know what your muscles feel when this happens? Hold your breath for as long as you possibly can.

➤ **Exercise lubricates your joints.** With decreased movement, the fluid surrounding your joints stops flowing. (Think Tin Man in *The Wizard of Oz*.) As we've said, movement encourages flow. Hence the stiff-legged, balky back gait you see from people walking down the aisle after a three-hour movie. Physiologically speaking, your joints are dry. Once you move, synovial fluid begins to flow again and it's easier for you to walk.

➤ **Exercise provides you with more energy.** Movement increases blood flow, removing waste products and delivering oxygen. Exercise also stimulates the release of feel-good hormones known as endorphins.

➤ **Exercise makes you look good!** Whoever invented the mirror probably knew that *Homo sapiens* are vain. Regular exercise is the best way we know to improve you appearance. Not only will you lose weight, your skin is apt to look better and your muscles will grow tauter. Know this: Feeling good about the way you look is highly contagious.

Yes, energy has both psychological and physical components. If you need to keep up with a boundless two-year old, there is no better way to do so than to get in a short workout or two during the day.

How Can 15, 30, or 60 Minutes Be Enough?

Why do short workouts make sense? Short workouts work for you when they fulfill the following two requirements:

➤ Effective.

➤ Efficient.

Still wed to the too-busy excuse? Let's say you only have 30 minutes between big meetings. Clear your head and strengthen your heart and legs by going for a brisk walk. Heading back to the office? A stair workout is probably one of the most effective and efficient exercises if you're on a tight schedule. And there are always trees to climb—though that may cause your coworkers to whisper behind your back.

Got 40 minutes? Walk for 25 minutes and then spend the next 10 minutes doing push-ups and crunches. Use the last five minutes to stretch. Just think of all the exercise possibilities you can do with an hour.

If your day is so busy that you're literally running from one meeting to the next, then consider the following:

➤ Take the stairs.

➤ Walk instead of taking a car or public transportation (you'll probably get there faster).

➤ Ride your bike or jog to and from work.

When you integrate exercise into your life, the possibilities are endless.

The Least You Need to Know

➤ You can find time for short workouts.

➤ Exercise does wonders to alleviate stress.

➤ Short workouts are the best way to maintain an exercise routine, especially if it's new.

➤ Short workouts provide you with both psychological and physical benefits.

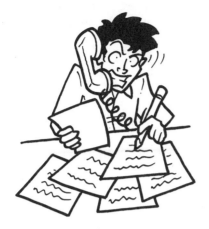

Chapter 2

Fitting It In

In This Chapter

➤ Time management tips for busy people

➤ A good excuse is usually just that

➤ Morning, noon, and evening workouts

➤ Exercise on the go

Even when you can't wrestle the time to go to the gym to do your full workout, you'll find that a short workout can do a world of good—making you more alert and relaxed throughout the day. In addition, by keeping active you avoid any setbacks in your fitness program. So while a 15-minute workout isn't enough to make huge improvements in your fitness (unless, of course, you've been inactive for a while), it can prevent any "detraining" effects. Plus if your goal is to lose weight, burning a few extra calories never hurts.

Often people say they don't have enough time when in fact what they lack more of is energy and willpower. Don't get us wrong: We're sympathetic to the demands of a busy life. But we've stood in the catbird seat countless times and seen that the same busy people who can't find 30 minutes to work out, spend an hour a day checking their e-mail, talking on the telephone, and/or watching TV and playing solitaire on the computer. If you think you don't have the time, think again. You can make it work if you just make some adjustments in your daily habits. And while it sounds a bit dramatic, it's crucial to know that if you don't work out now, you're likely to pay for it later.

In this chapter we'll provide you with tips on detecting just how much time you are wasting as well as ways to develop successful time-management habits.

Excuses, Excuses

Before we continue, let's see if any of the following reasons for not working out sounds familiar:

➤ I have to work late tonight.

➤ I've got to pick up the kids.

➤ I have to make dinner.

➤ I travel so much for my job I can't stick to a workout routine.

➤ I spend so much time working I don't want to spend my free time working out.

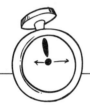

Short Cuts

What we find again and again is that people who make the effort to squeeze in a quickie workout begin to crave the buzz that vigorous exercise supplies. Once people learn to make working out part of their weekly routine, the "can't find time" dragon is slain.

Free time? What's free time? We're here to tell you that you don't have to spend every bit of your leisure time exercising and that you can have positive results with as little as 15 minutes a pop. Armed with the knowledge that exercise—any exercise—can energize you and make you more productive during the day makes people more motivated to do even the shortest of workouts.

Therein lies the rub: If you lack the energy to work out, you're less likely to get to the gym or do an at-home workout. However, once you get to the gym or your exercise equipment in your TV room (isn't that where you keep your Stairmaster?), you'll see that you have more energy. What will get you over the hump? Willpower and the belief that you don't have to workout like an aspiring Olympian to improve your fitness. And, as we've already stressed, finding activities you enjoy is crucial.

Time Management

There's a great expression, "If you want to get something done, give it to a busy person." While that's probably true, if you are busy the only way to remain productive is to be organized. In fact, the busier you are, the more organized you have to be if you want to keep body and soul together. The catch-22 here is that often people who think they're busy assume they have less time because they're poorly organized. We all know people who spend much of their time sifting through papers in search for their to-do list. (The first item was undoubtedly "straighten up desk.")

There are, of course, different ways to skin a cat. Witness this goofy example: While writing *The Complete Idiot's Guide to Weight Training*, it became increasingly clear that the husband-and-wife team of Deidre and Jonathan have very different styles of organization. Jonathan is Oscar Madison: papers scattered all over, books piled on his desk and around his chair like a minifortress. (Deidre calls it a disaster area; Jonathan considers it a sign of high intelligence.) While Jonathan's personalized system looks chaotic, he knows which end is up and is very efficient at organizing and prioritizing. On the other hand, Deidre, the Felix Unger of this odd couple, cannot tell you her middle name if her pencils aren't sharpened and facing in the same direction. The bottom line is that while no one way is perfect, you need to be organized if you want to get things done.

Still dubious? Here are some ways to help you manage your time more effectively:

➤ Plan a week at a time, keeping your long-term priorities in mind. Considering the many hats you may have to wear in the course of the day (not to mention the various goals you have), it's easy to get distracted and lose your focus. By planning for the entire week, you can factor in your multiple roles and goals and get things done.

➤ Make a to-do list with no more than seven key items. Assign a letter of priority to each item on your list: *A* for must do first, *B* for should do after *A*, *C* for must get done but not necessarily today, and so forth. Cross each out when completed and make a new list of your top goals.

➤ Keep your written goals where you can see them—and not under a pile of papers on your desk. Seeing them is like having a benevolent drill sergeant at your side so you stay on track.

➤ Just say "no"! Essentially, this means prioritizing your needs. Participate in a few key activities and politely decline others.

➤ Stop trying to be perfect, when you don't have to be. Instead of taking tons of time writing the perfect thank-you note to your Aunt Tilly, jot down a quick heartfelt card or note. When leaving a message with a friend or business associate that doesn't need a reply, call after hours and leave a message on his answering machine.

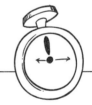

Short Cuts

Combine tasks so you can do more than one thing at a time. Before you know it you've freed up valuable hours in your cramped day.

While all of these tips sound good in theory, let's give you a few day-to-day tactics to illustrate just what we're talking about.

➤ If you take a lunch to work, make it the night before. This will give you more time in the morning to get the children ready for their day.

➤ If you have school-age children, make their lunch the night before.

➤ To leave more time in the morning, lay out the clothes you plan to wear the night before. (Make sure you listen to the weather report.)

➤ Bring work-related reading material with you when you're running errands. If you're on a long line at the supermarket, for example, whip it out and read while you wait.

➤ Establish routines with regular chores like paying your bills. This way you won't fall behind (which means paying extra) and it won't absorb much of your mental energy.

The key to time management is learning how to reorganize your life so that you have some stress-free time to exercise.

Finding the Time

If you still think you don't have time to fit exercise into your already scheduled life, please do the following written exercise. For one week, record the amount of time you spend on the following activities.

Activity	Minutes	Hours
Nonwork-related phone calls	_____	_____
Watching television	_____	_____
Daydreaming	_____	_____
Listening to the radio	_____	_____
Playing on the computer	_____	_____
Eating out	_____	_____
Schmoozing with neighbors who dropped by to say "hello"	_____	_____
Hanging out with your friends after work	_____	_____
TOTAL TIME	_____	_____

At the end of a week, add up the amount of time that you spent on the above activities and odds are that you could squeeze in a few hour-long workouts at the gym.

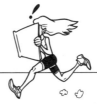

Info to Go

The average American watches more than four hours of TV each day. At this rate, by age 65, that person will have spent nine years of his or her life watching television (or 28 hours per week, two months of nonstop TV watching per year).

While many people think that getting organized means they have to become rigid, the reality is that discipline and order help you become more free. No longer must you burn tons of mental energy holding on to idle fantasies that you never acted on. If you're able to manage your time effectively, you'll be surprised at how easy it is to get things done as well as the added time you'll have to just do nothing.

The eight activities listed above are rather obvious ways that we waste time. However, according to Warren Wint, who runs Total Success Training, a London-based management consulting firm, other copious time wasters include the following:

➤ Indecision and procrastination. If you are unsure about how a task should be done and feel silly about asking, you are more likely to continue to put it on the back burner until you are forced to come to grips with it.

➤ Tasks you do that you should have delegated. The manager who takes the minutes at office meetings, types them, and makes copies of them for distribution in addition to other duties is not making the most of his or her time.

➤ Acting on a project without sufficient information. If you don't understand the exact purpose or meaning of the project, you are apt to make a mistake that would require more time to correct.

➤ Unclear information. If you don't understand what you are supposed to do and you do it wrong, you'll have to do it all over again. Get the facts before you start.

➤ Lack of planning. Literally, think about what you want to do before you do it. Plot it out and consider any and all possibilities.

➤ Stress and fatigue. When you are under stress and are fatigued, your thinking becomes cloudy and your ability to make good clear decisions is compromised.

➤ Inability to say no. Stretching yourself too thin can result in poor execution of projects.

➤ Personal disorganization. Spending most of your time looking for papers and other assorted items can be a colossal waste of time.

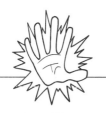

Stop Short

To live a fitness lifestyle, change from a sedentary lifestyle is essential. The key, however, is to seek small changes, not big end points. Once your weekly workout pattern is established, (usually after about eight weeks) the hardest part of the battle has been won.

When Jonathan sets up exercise programs for clients new to exercise, he stresses that the most important thing they can do over the first few weeks is make exercise part of their daily routine. He asks them about their daily routine and helps them integrate fitness into their day.

During those precious first few weeks, he's far more concerned with them developing that habit than with the particular exercises they do. The key is getting people to show up at the gym. Even if all you do is talk about Lance Armstrong's win at the Tour de France or the last great movie you saw, he's satisfied that you've begun to integrate working out into your daily routine.

If you work out at home, make a promise to yourself that you're going to find time to work out. Often writing in your daily planner that you must work out is all the commitment you need. You can reward yourself by popping in a video to watch as you spin on your stationary bike. If, however, you realize that you're not getting the job done on your own, think seriously about joining a gym, running club, or some other organized fitness group.

By now we assume that we've convinced you that working out for an hour or less is enough to help you improve your fitness. Now let's figure out when you're going to find the time.

For Early Birds Only

There's an old expression that goes something like: "An hour in the morning is worth two in the evening." In other words, working out in the morning is a great time to exercise—assuming you're able to wake up and get out the door. It's quiet, there's less traffic if you ride your bike or drive to the gym, and it's a great way to organize your thoughts for the day ahead. After a good workout and shower, you're bound to head to work feeling energized and virtuous at the same time. That way, no matter how busy you get later in the day, your workout is in the books. If the morning seems like a good time slot for you, consider the following to make it easier.

When Deidre was winning national power-lifting championships, she was also a full-time student in physical therapy school and working a part-time job. Needless to say, she was pressed for time and had no choice but to work out in the wee hours of the morning. Here are her early morning workout tips.

1. Listen to the weather forecast and lay out your clothes for both work and working out the night before. That way you won't have to rush around looking for your favorite shorts and matching socks.

2. If you take your lunch to work, make it the night before. Don't forget to take it out of the fridge when you leave in the morning.

3. Lose the snooze button. One wake-up call is all you get.

4. A coffeemaker with a timer is often a good get-out-of-bed incentive.

5. Put your feet on the floor before your mate smashes the alarm clock or sabotages your incentive to stick to your exercise program.

If you live within walking/jogging distance from work, a great way to commute and work out at the same time is to hoof it to work. Jonathan, who loves cycling far more than running, often jogs to work with his work clothes in a backpack a few times a week instead of taking the subway. (He dislikes crowded subways more than he does running.)

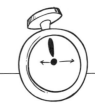

Considering that the ride on the train takes only five minutes more than the run, the time commitment is virtually the same. If you don't have the luxury of working in shorts and a T-shirt like Jonathan, you can carry a week's worth of work clothes in a garment bag every Monday and change at the office. Of course, without access to a shower you're bound to alienate even the most tolerant of your co-workers.

Another good idea assuming that you belong to a gym near your job is to run to the gym in the morning. If you have extra time, you can lift weights and stretch there before you shower. Most gyms offer rental lockers, so you can keep all your toiletries there.

Short Cuts

Prework workouts are great if you have some exercise equipment at home. In Chapter 6, "Strengthening," we'll give you some ideas for setting up a home gym without sapping your bank account or crowding your space.

Don't like running? Cycling is a practical alternative to driving or taking mass transportation. (Often it's faster.) According to the August 2000 issue of *Bicycling* magazine, commuting 15 miles, three times per week, can save $271 in depreciation on your car and save you more than $7,000 in gas, insurance, and car payments. Factor in about 40,000 calories burned and you're way ahead of the game.

How About Lunch?

Lunchtime is a great opportunity to take a step away from your busy day in order to get in a quick workout. Not only will you be physically rejuvenated for the rest of the day, you're likely to work with a clearer head as well. However, working out during lunch is tricky and you have to be extremely focused and organized.

The toughest part about a midday workout is making sure you have enough to eat to prevent you from getting hungry once you're back at work. The best way to do that is to bring food with you to work so you can eat throughout the morning and early afternoon. This is called grazing and it's really the best way to eat, as long as you are eating healthful foods such as fruits, raw veggies, nuts, and yogurt. Once you're back at the office from your workout, you can eat a turkey sandwich or a tuna sandwich.

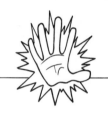

Stop Short

Keep in mind that lunch is the meal when many people's diets come undone. Unlike meals that you prepare at home, you usually have less control over what you eat when you dine out. Take a look at Chapter 4, "Nutrition," for nutrition tips when you eat out.

Here are some criteria for working out during lunch:

➤ Make sure the health club is near your job. You don't want to spend 20 minutes of your lunch hour traveling.

➤ Take a class (spinning, aerobic, step, toning). The great thing about a lunchtime class is that it'll be geared to people like you with no time to spare. Odds are they'll be sure to get you back to your desk in under an hour.

➤ Look for a club that provides amenities such as soap, shampoo, and towels. This saves you the trouble of having to lug these things with you.

Even if you don't have access to a gym during lunch or a full hour to spare, try to do some physical activity, since some is better than none. Don't have your lunch delivered if you can take a walk to go get it instead. Take a short break and stretch for a few minutes. Breathing fresh air will leave you more alert and ready to do your best work.

After Work Workouts

While some of us are ready for nothing more ambitious than watching the evening news after work, there are plenty of people who get their second wind once they leave the office. If this is the best workout time for your, here are some tips:

➤ If your gym is near your home, go straight there rather than heading home first. Once you open your own front door, there's a load of reasons for you to miss your workout. (Did anyone say nap?)

➤ Grab a snack such as a piece of fruit, pretzels, a nutrition bar, or another health-ful snack an hour or two before your workout. There's nothing worse than going to the gym hungry. You'll be distracted and less energetic.

➤ Of course, like our early birds that ran, skated, or cycled to work, you can do the same from your office to your home.

The bottom line is experimenting to see what works best for your body and schedule. If you pre-fer working out in the morning because you have more pep but have a friend who will run with you in the evening, try both and see which you prefer.

On the Run

Nothing interrupts a workout routine faster than lots of overtime and business travel. With a little dedication and planning for the unexpected, you can continue to work out while tending to life's surprises. Whether you're stuck at work or on the road, there are ways you can help manage your fit-ness goals.

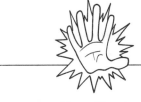

Stop Short

If you exercise outdoors after dark (or before sunrise), be sure to wear reflective clothing or wear a portable light on your body or bike.

Work Out at Work

When overtime beckons, you have to step up to the plate. Again, please heed our ral-lying cry that exercising for as little as 15 minutes at a time is beneficial. You can take several 15-minute breaks by doing the following:

➤ **Take a brisk walk.** It will burn a few calories, get your blood flowing, and clear your head. If you have to go to a meeting, consider walking instead of driving or using public transportation if you can.

➤ **Use the stairs.** Deidre usually hustles up the stairs in lieu of the elevator when she visits her patients. By the end of the day she's often totaled 50 flights.

➤ **Stretch.** There are lots of great stretches you can do at your desk. Check Chap-ter 22, "Five-Minute Workouts at the Office," for some ideas.

On the Road Again

People who have jobs that require a lot of travel face some of the biggest fitness hur-dles. In Chapter 21, "Working Out on the Road," we'll outline equipment—from rub-ber bands to jump ropes to water-filled dumbbells—that you can take on the road. (We'll also give you some workouts you can do while when you're on the road.)

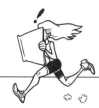

Info to Go

Running as transportation is "easier" and has a different feel than running purely for recreation. (Even if the results are the same.) Jonathan, who manages several fitness centers throughout New York City, regularly runs from site to site. While some of these jaunts take just a few minutes, the mental and physical benefits would be lost had he driven or taken public transportation.

Many gyms have national affiliations that allow you to use their facilities all over the country for a nominal fee. Even if you don't have a gym, we'll give you ideas of how to get a good workout on the road.

We've given you some ideas of how and when you can squeeze in a productive workout. Not convinced? In Chapter 5, "Aerobics," we'll outline all sorts of time management ideas that will help you free up the time that you need.

Setting Goals

Before any fitness professional promises you the moon, we want you to understand that everyone has a particular body type and genetic makeup that cannot be altered. This means that no matter how much you work out, if you are five foot two and 140 pounds, even dropping 20 pounds isn't going to make you look like a professional model. In fact, dropping that much weight is going to make you look like a fitter version of you. So don't set goals that are impossible to achieve. That's a prescription for failure and disappointment.

There are, of course, three specific fitness goals that you can set for yourself: to increase your cardiovascular fitness, your physical strength, and your flexibility. Below we will outline why you want to achieve these various fitness goals.

Why Develop Your Cardiovascular Fitness?

Too often, we think, people assume that being fit means lifting weights. While total fitness and toned muscles often go together, strength training alone is just one piece of the workout puzzle. Another key component is your ticker—cardiovascular fitness to you sophisticated types. The benefits are obvious and many.

➤ To achieve and maintain weight loss.

➤ To reduce and maintain healthy cholesterol levels.

➤ To reduce the risk of heart disease.

➤ To manage high blood pressure.

➤ To reduce tension and control stress.

➤ To reduce anxiety and depression.

➤ To boost your energy level.

➤ To keep up with your kids.

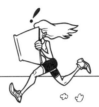

Info to Go

According to Steve Ilg, a personal trainer that *Outside* magazine labeled one of the fittest men on earth: "Your body is a masterpiece, intricate in function, unique in its mix of attributes and abilities. Give praise—you are wonderfully, singularly made!" So while it's fine to aspire to look like an Olympic swimmer, don't despair if you fall short of your expectation. Remember that the athletes who make it to the Olympics are blessed with great genes and an incredible work ethic.

Why Build Up Your Physical Strength?

Conversely, we know plenty of runners and cyclists who have done so much cardio training that their heart beats only on the weekends. We applaud their efforts; however, there are just as many reasons to add a bit of strength training to their regime as there are for strength-training devotees to improve their cardio fitness.

➤ To increase your lean body mass, which helps you burn more calories at rest.

➤ To prevent bone loss, which can begin in your 30s.

➤ To reduce tension and control stress.

➤ To improve your self-image.

➤ Easier pregnancy and delivery. Quicker recovery postpregnancy to prepregnancy shape.

➤ To help you accomplish physical tasks such as carrying the baby carriage up the stairs or groceries home from the supermarket.

➤ To help you age gracefully. We begin to lose muscle mass in the third decade of life at a rate of about one pound of muscle each year or 8 percent per decade. It's no wonder that the elderly are virtual prisoners in their own homes, often unable to stand without assistance, clean, or shop.

Why Extend Your Flexibility?

Stretching is probably the most neglected aspect of working out. Why? Because, first, it's hard, especially if you're tight. Second, many people don't feel as if they're doing anything. We're sympathetic to both concerns, but trust us when we say that stretching regularly is essential, especially when those grey hairs start appearing. Here's why:

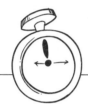

Short Cuts

Don't weigh yourself every day—it only leads to frustration since your weight fluctuates throughout the day. (For women, throughout the month as well.) Try weighing yourself at the same time and on the same day of the week once a week. We usually tip the scales first thing every Monday morning.

➤ To prevent injury to tight muscles that are not properly warmed up.

➤ To maintain muscular balance. What does that mean? Imagine sitting at your desk in that typical forward slouched position. The muscles in the front part of your body become contracted and tight, which in the long term can lead to permanent postural changes (like the upper back hump that the elderly get).

➤ To continue being able to perform normal, daily tasks like reaching up in the cupboard for dishes.

➤ To continue being able to scratch your back yourself.

➤ To continue being able to give yourself a pedicure if you are on a budget.

With proper diet and exercise you can be the best physical specimen that your particular genetic make-up allows you to be. Your goal should not be to look like the actresses or models that peer out at us from every magazine cover and poster. Base your goals on your own desires—a smaller dress or pants size, to be stronger or more flexible. These are goals that are tangible and will keep you interested and motivated.

Values-Based Prioritizing

Values-based prioritizing may sound complicated, but it's really just another way of saying that you decide which aspect of fitness is the most important for you at the time. Is it weight loss? Cardiovascular fitness? Are you eager to get stronger? Once you set your goals, we can help you design a workout stacked in that direction.

In the chapters to follow we'll give you specific routines that you can do to make your fitness goals a reality even if you're pressed for time.

The Least You Need to Know

➤ Time management is an important tool in being effective and productive.

➤ You can plot your time to determine how much is spent doing nonproductive activities.

➤ Success with your fitness regimen requires making it a priority.

➤ Base your workout routine on your personal fitness goals.

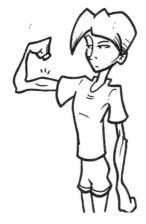

Chapter 3

Workouts and Your Body

> **In This Chapter**
>
> ➤ Assessing your fitness goals
>
> ➤ Exercising with asthma, hypertension, and diabetes
>
> ➤ Figuring out what your level of fitness is
>
> ➤ Debunking a few myths

Before we get to the nitty-gritty of working out, let's step back and assess the status of your current health and fitness. While we agree that this isn't an overly exciting topic, it is important. As a result, this chapter will discuss the basics of getting a clean bill of health from your doctor as well as questions that relate to specific medical concerns. The good news is that very few medical conditions should prevent you from working out.

Once we've established what you need to know before you start, we'll help you figure out what your exercise options are, how to measure your current level of fitness, and how your body responds to working out. Equally important, we'll tell you how it responds when you miss workouts.

What's Up, Doc?

Clearly if you're a member of the U.S. Olympic team, able to leap tall buildings in a single bound, or under the legal drinking age, you can start a new exercise program without a physical. However, if you've been inactive for a while, recently ill, or have a specific medical issue, it's a very good idea to see a physician for a checkup. Remember, even if you do have a health problem, there are plenty of exercise options available; however, a little knowledge will give you more confidence as well as make your workouts safer and more productive.

If you'd rather not get a physical, at the very least you should take a look at the Physical Activity Readiness Questionnaire (PAR Q), a chart developed by the Canadian Society for Exercise Physiology. This nifty screening tool was designed for anyone between the ages of 15 and 69 and should give you an idea of where you stand.

Use PAR Q as a screening tool before you start an exercise program.

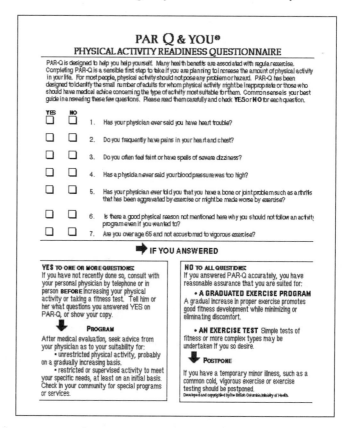

Look at the PAR Q. If you honestly answered no to each of the questions, then according to the PAR Q it's fine for you to get started. Although, to state the obvious, even if you've just completed an Ironman triathlon, start a new regime slowly and build up gradually.

If you answered "yes" to any of the questions or are over 70, you should definitely check with your doctor. As we said, it's unlikely that exercise will be nixed, but you should get the okay first.

Now let's take a look at some of the most common medical conditions that need to be addressed.

Hypertension

Hypertension, or high blood pressure, affects about 50 million Americans. For most people with mild to moderate hypertension, exercise is one of the most effective treatments. And though many doctors won't rush to tell you this, a regular exercise program can help you decrease or entirely eliminate medication. Here's why. When you do aerobic exercise your blood vessels dilate—and remain dilated even after you stop. That causes your blood pressure (BP) to decrease. (One of the most common categories of BP medications is vasodilators, so as we said, exercise could have the same effect as medication.) While it's generally safe for people with hypertension to lift weights, it's especially important not to lift real heavy weights. When you "max out," you tend to hold your breath. This is known as the Valsalva maneuver to us physio types, and it's quite dangerous for anyone with high blood pressure.

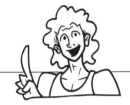

Workout Words

Hypertension is defined as a resting blood pressure of 140/90 or greater. Textbook "normal" pressure is 120/80, though there's no need to worry if it's a little higher. The top figure, or systolic pressure corresponds to the pressure as your heart contracts, while the lower number, or diastolic pressure is the pressure as your heart relaxes between beats.

Diabetes

Diabetes is a condition in which an insufficient amount of insulin (the hormone necessary for the metabolism of blood sugar/blood glucose) is produced by the body. Under normal conditions insulin is released to counteract the increased blood sugar that comes after a meal. If you have Type I or juvenile onset diabetes, the body typically doesn't release enough insulin. Those with Type II, or adult onset diabetes, tend to be resistant to insulin, which means insulin doesn't do what it supposed to.

Because exercise has an "insulin-like" effect, your doctor needs to know if you are diabetic and beginning an exercise program. This is important because your doctor may adjust the timing of your medications. And, in the case of insulin, change where you make your injections. (Injecting an exercising muscle is likely to increase the rate of absorption.)

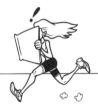

Info to Go

If you're diagnosed with diabetes and worried about not reaching your full athletic potential, know that three of the best athletes of the twentieth century—Ty Cobb (baseball), Arthur Ashe (tennis), and Joe Frazier (boxing)—were athletes who managed diabetes.

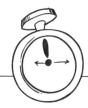

Short Cuts

A review by University Hospital in Antwerp, Belgium, has found that moderate weight loss is more likely to be maintained over time. Setting an attainable goal helps you stick with your exercise program. Plus, if your blood pressure is high, modest exercise will help normalize it even if it takes longer to reach your ideal weight. Reducing your weight only 5 percent to 10 percent may also reduce your risk of cardiovascular disease, Type II diabetes, and the need to take medications for your blood pressure.

There is a host of do's and don'ts that diabetics need to become familiar with:

1. Weight loss and modifications in your diet can play a large role for people with adult onset diabetes.

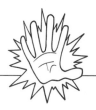

Stop Short

It's a good idea for diabetics to carry a piece of candy with them while they exercise in case of a hypoglycemic episode.

2. If you have adult onset diabetes, it's important—no matter how busy your day becomes—that you don't let too much time pass between meals. (Skipping meals is a real no-no.) In order to stabilize your blood sugar, it's important that your carbohydrate intake as well as the timing of your meals remain consistent. Again, talk to your doctor or a nutritionist for more info.

3. It sounds odd, but diabetics are advised to wear good socks and sneakers and carefully check their feet for cuts or blisters because of a condition known as diabetic neuropathy. As a result, diabetics occasionally have decreased sensation in their feet and can therefore be unaware of damage.

Asthma

Many of us think of asthmatics as woefully frail sickly people who double over when they run up a flight of stairs. Well, consider Olympic gold medallist Jackie Joyner-Kersee, a heptathlete who is arguably the greatest female athlete of our time. Our poster boy for dealing with this tough condition, Jonathan Cane, has done 150 bicycle races over the past five years and, for the record, has raced up the stairs of the Empire State Building four times. In other words, asthma does not need to prevent you from working out. Asthma medications have come a long way in the past few years, and most are very effective and free of side effects. (Although it's quite possible that one of the lesser-known side effects is an irrational need to sprint up stairwells in skyscrapers. If this happens more than once, please have your doctor adjust your medication.)

As Jonathan has learned firsthand, asthma sufferers may want to avoid exercising in cold and dry conditions. If you're working out and find that the cold air is bothering you, often breathing through your nose helps filter and warm the air before it hits your lungs.

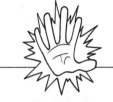

Stop Short

If you have asthma, it's real important for you to warm up thoroughly before any aerobic activity. The gradual increase helps prevent attacks.

Measuring Your Fitness Level

Think of someone getting in the car and driving aimlessly without a map, directions, or destination. This might be a good agenda if you're checking how many miles to the gallon your car gets, but otherwise it's a good way to get nowhere fast. In short, that's the mistake many people we see make—novices and seasoned veterans alike. Sure, it's great that you're in the gym, but without a specific plan it's surprisingly difficult to make real progress. Here are two important points to consider:

1. What are your goals? Do you want to get stronger? Improve your sports performance? Your appearance? Are you trying to lose weight or gain muscle? Improve your ability to carry the baby stroller up the stairs or are you in the gym to improve your 10K time?

2. Where do you stand today? How fit are you? How flexible? What about muscular strength and cardiovascular endurance? What's your percentage of body fat? (Aren't you glad we've begun to thoroughly confuse you?) By clearly defining your goals and establishing your current state of fitness, you can have a direction to your training and measure the progress that you make. Remember, even the most brilliant architect follows a plan.

Each of us has different goals and no single goal is right or wrong. If the only motivation you have for working out is to look good in a bathing suit, no worries. If you're a racer like Jonathan and Joe who head to the gym to enhance their cycling and marathon kayaking performances, you'll be spending a fair bit of time doing specific exercises geared toward that goal. (Although Joe won't admit it, he's been considering paddling this season in a pink Speedo.) When Deidre competed as a power lifter, she focused on her three primary lifts. Now that's she's retired and spends a lot of time polishing her trophies, her gym workouts have virtually nothing to do with lifting small buildings and everything to do with looking and feeling good.

The good news, of course, is there's plenty of overlap. The runner, who lifts to get faster on the road, inevitably winds up looking better before and after the race. The person who trains like a Trojan to squeeze into the tiniest bathing suit possible each summer will, on a good exercise regime, wind up having more energy to play with her kids and be better able to run through the airport with her luggage to catch a plane.

While you need to know where you're going, it's also valuable to find out where you're at. You can do this in a variety of ways. The best is to go to a lab, fitness center, or physiology department at a university and have some number-crunching physiologists like Jonathan poke and prod you to measure your cardiovascular fitness, muscular strength and endurance, flexibility, and body composition. If you know where you can get tested, we strongly suggest that you take advantage of them. If you don't have a qualified professional to perform these tests, there are still benchmarks that you can test yourself. (Of course you can call Jonathan, but he might ride his bike there and that gets time consuming.) If you live in the Australian outback or just can't be bothered, here are a few measurements you can take to gauge your own fitness.

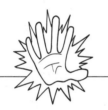

Stop Short

Heart rate can also be measured at the carotid artery in the neck, but we recommend that you stick to the radial pulse in the wrist. If you press too hard on your neck it can cause a reflexive decrease in your heart rate and cause you to become dizzy or faint.

Resting Heart Rate

The first thing you should do is monitor your resting heart rate. The best time to do this is first thing in the morning—after you use the bathroom since having to go may otherwise elevate your heart rate. Here's what to do.

1. Place your index and middle fingers together on the opposite wrist, about half an inch on the inside of the joint, in line with the index finger.

2. Feel for a pulse by pressing lightly on the artery.

3. Once you find a strong pulse, count the number of beats you feel for one minute.

4. Begin your count with zero. When exercising, it's more practical to take your heart rate for 10 seconds and multiply by six.

Knowing your resting heart rate does not necessarily tell you much—it's a number relative to nothing—but noting changes over time generally indicates a change in your level of fitness. As your heart and cardiovascular system becomes stronger and more efficient, your resting heart rate (RHR) will decrease. This indicates that more blood is being pumped with each beat and that your body is more efficient at extracting oxygen from the blood.

Often we're asked, "What's a good normal resting heart rate?" That's a good question with no real answer. Normal RHR ranges from 60 to 100 beats per minute; the average is approximately 70 for men and 75 for women. Extremely well-conditioned athletes sometimes have heart rates as low as 40 beats per minute. Former tennis great Bjorn Borg was said to have a RHR around 36 beats per minute.

Weight and Body Composition

The "Body Mass Index" (BMI) is a quick way to gauge if you're at a healthy weight. But because it does not differentiate between muscle and fat, or take frame size into account, it is clearly a flawed method. However, for someone who isn't extremely muscular, it's a reasonably accurate and quick method. High BMIs—the bane of many American's existence—are associated with an increase risk of heart disease, hypertension, and diabetes. Here's a chart to look up your BMI:

Body Mass Index

Weight Category	BMI Range	% Above
Normal weight	19–25	
Overweight	26–30	20–40%
Obese	31–35	41–100%
Seriously obese	Over 35	Over 100%

Regardless of what the scale says, the best way to determine if you need to lose weight is by measuring your body composition. That's because body composition measurements take your muscle mass in to account and can differentiate between a lean, mean bodybuilder who's covered in muscle and weighs 210 pounds and a couch potato with a gut who's the same height and weight.

There are a variety of tests available in lab settings: Underwater weighing is the gold standard, and skin-fold calipers are dependable and reliable. Other methods such as bioelectrical impedence are impressive looking (and sounding) but notoriously inaccurate. If you don't have access to those tests, here's a quick test you can do to *estimate* your body fat percentage.

1. Measure your height in inches.
2. Measure the widest part of your hips in inches.
3. Using the chart, take a straight edge and match up each end to your corresponding height and hip girth. The point at which the ruler intersects the middle line is your estimated percent body fat.

Use this chart to estimate the percentage of body fat you carry.

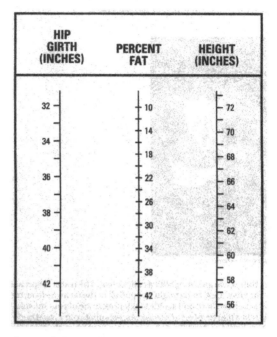

Muscular Strength and Endurance

Push-ups—that simplest of exercises used by drill sergeants and gym teachers—are a good way to test your upper-body strength quickly and easily. Women should use a modified push-up, with their knees bent and on the floor, and men should keep their toes on the floor with legs out straight.

Start at the top position with your arms straight and lower yourself until your chest is about a clenched fist's distance from the floor. Keep your back straight throughout. See how many you can do without breaking form or resting at the top or bottom. Test yourself every few months to measure the progress of your strength routine. Below are norms so that you can check yourself against other in your age category.

Push-Up Norms for Men

Age	20–29	30–39	40–49	50–59	60+
Excellent	55+	44+	40+	35+	30+
Good	45–54	35–44	30–39	25–34	20–29
Average	35–44	25–34	20–29	15–24	10–19
Fair	20–34	15–24	12–19	8–14	5–9
Low	0–19	0–14	0–11	0–7	0–4

Push-Up Norms for Women

Age	20–29	30–39	40–49	50–59	60+
Excellent	49+	40+	35+	30+	20+
Good	34–48	25–39	20–34	15–29	5–19
Average	17–33	12–24	8–19	6–14	3–4
Fair	6–16	4–11	3–7	2–5	1–2
Low	0–5	0–3	0–2	0–1	0

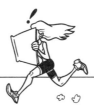

Info to Go

To some people, the standard test of strength is the one-rep-max bench press. While some folks like to do maximal tests for strength, we see no reason to take the risk. There's a much higher incidence of injury in attempts to lift as much as possible for one rep, so unless you're a competitive power lifter, there's no justification. It doesn't matter how strong you are if you're on the disabled list with a shoulder injury or a pulled pectoral muscle.

Cardiovascular Tests

Again, there is no replacement for the testing available in a lab, but there are a few you can do on your own to estimate your cardiovascular fitness.

A simple yet arduous test, widely used in the military and law-enforcement agencies, is the 1.5-mile walk/run. The procedure is simple:

1. Find a treadmill, quarter-mile track, or another accurately measured, flat 1.5-mile course.
2. After a thorough warm-up, run and/or walk 1.5 miles as fast as possible.

Here are the norms for men and women, broken down by 10-year age groups.

Women's Norms per Age Group

Rank	20–29	30–39	40–49	50–59	60+
Superior	10:47	11:49	12:51	14:20	14:06
Excellent	12:51	13:43	14:31	15:57	16:20
Good	14:24	15:08	15:57	16:58	17:46
Fair	15:26	15:57	16:58	17:55	18:44
Poor	16:33	17:14	18:00	18:49	19:21
Very Poor	18:14	18:31	19:05	19:57	20:23

Men's Norms per Age Group

Rank	20–29	30–39	40–49	50–59	60+
Superior	8:13	8:44	9:30	10:40	11:20
Excellent	10:16	10:47	11:44	12:51	13:53
Good	11:41	12:20	13:14	14:24	15:29
Fair	12:51	13:36	14:29	15:26	16:43
Poor	14:13	14:52	15:41	16:43	18:00
Very Poor	16:12	16:27	17:23	18:31	20:04

Flexibility

We're constantly amazed how many strong and "fit" men we see in the gym who are unable to touch their toes. This begs the question: Can you be truly fit if you're as flexible as an elephant's tusk?

The most common test used by physiologists to measure flexibility is known as the "sit-and-reach" test. This is basically a seated toe touch using a specially designed box to measure how far forward you bend. The test is valuable because poor performance usually indicates the likelihood of lower-back injury.

Odds are you don't have a sit-and-reach box at home, but you can still get a basic idea of your lower back, hip, and hamstring flexibility. Try this. In your bare feet, sit on the floor with your feet six inches apart and flat against the wall. Bend forward slowly, without bouncing. If you can easily touch the wall, your flexibility is fine. If you can barely reach the wall, it's fair. If you can't reach the wall (don't cheat and bend your knees), jog to your nearest yoga teacher. Actually, walk; you might pull a hamstring otherwise.

Looking Good

As we mentioned earlier, if your main motivation for exercise is looking good, fret not. A good body usually means that you're on the right track. Just as important, looking good is good for your mind. Having someone say he thought you were 5 or 10 years younger than you are is a simple yet satisfying pleasure. And appearing younger than your peers is also great for your self-confidence as well.

Feeling Healthy

It sounds simple, but people who exercise usually take better care of themselves. When you're committed to working out, it becomes a part of your life and begins to influence many small decisions you make throughout the day. Will you have ice cream for a snack or a piece of fruit instead? Will you have the chicken Parmesan or the spaghetti with marinara sauce? For dessert, will you have the Mississippi Mud Cake or the fruit custard?

After a while, you will begin to notice how much better you feel with more healthful food choices. What you'll also realize is that the better you eat, the more energy you have at work, play, or working out. You've heard of vicious cycles? Well, this is a good "vicious" cycle that you want to initiate.

Here's an important point that turns many people off. Eating better doesn't mean you have to swear off ice cream or filet mignon. What we are saying is that with exercise and healthful eating, you'll feel so good that you will want to make the major indulgences a minor part of your life.

Being Strong

We know we don't have to convince men that being strong is a good thing, since the male psyche seems to relish the role strength plays in life. Women, however, are a different story. Many women equate being strong with having "bulky" muscles. (Not that there is anything wrong with that.) Simply put, this is a misconception that keeps many women from lifting weights in the first place. Those that do lift, often use weights that are so light you'd need to do 9,000 repetitions to get the full effect. (For the record: Three sets of 9,000 take about eight hours.)

Below are some myths about women and strength, and the facts that set the record straight.

Myth 1: Being Strong Means Having Big Muscles

Strength and muscularity are not the same. Strength is the ability to resist force or strain. Muscularity is the ability to develop mass and has to do with your genetic make-up. Huh? We all have a genetic code that determines everything from the color of our eyes to the length of our legs. The size of our muscles is also determined by the genetics passed along by our parents. This is why you can have a guy who looks like a fire truck who can't lift as much weight as a lean, wiry guy built like a greyhound. Why? Because Mr. Fire Truck has the genetics for big muscles and Mr. Greyhound does not.

Myth 2: Heavy Weights and Low Reps Give You Bulk; Light Weights and High Reps Give Your Muscles That Long, Lean Look

Again, the shape and size of your muscles is genetically predetermined. Whether you perform biceps curls with 20 pounds for 10 repetitions, or 10 pounds for 20 repetitions, your muscles will look the way they are wired to look.

Myth 3: Lifting Weights Makes Women Look Muscle-Bound

This is a little hard to answer because it depends on what your definition of muscle-bound is. If you are thinking about the superpumped women on the cover of *Muscle & Fitness,* don't worry about it unless you have a testosterone level equal to Arnold Schwarzenegger (and a steroid level equal to that of a well-medicated racehorse). Achieving any level of muscularity requires long-term dedication—a level of time and energy that most people don't have. In other words, going to the gym three times a week to strength train is not going to make you any more "muscle-bound" than running on the treadmill several times a week will make you an Olympic-level marathoner.

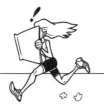

Info to Go

An inactive 60-year-old will lose 25 percent to 30 percent of the muscle mass she had at age 30. This can lead to decreased mobility, slowed metabolism, and an increase in the chance of getting injured.

Fortunately, being strong does not require you to look like Ms. Olympia and the benefits are well worth putting in the time.

Not only can increased muscle and strength help you perform better on and off the court, it can have practical benefits as well. Deidre, a physical therapist who works with many elderly patients, finds that many of her clients are unable to do things that we take for granted. Things like going grocery shopping alone, doing laundry, and even getting in and out of the shower. Many of these people are forced to hire aides to help them with normal activities of daily life, making them virtual prisoners in their own homes. Often such dependence is the result of years of neglect. This is reason enough to begin participating in a strengthening routine.

How Your Body Responds to Exercise

While virtually everyone knows that working out makes you look and feel good, not that many know how and why. What happens physiologically when you exercise?

Let's look at how your body responds to different types of exercise.

Cardiovascular Exercise

Your cardiovascular system is made up of your heart, lungs, and blood vessels. With continued exercise, your cardiovascular system becomes stronger and more efficient.

As we mentioned earlier, as your heart becomes stronger, it is capable of ejecting more blood with each beat. (This is known as your stroke volume.) This means that your heart doesn't have to beat as often. In addition, your lung capacity increases and your muscles are capable of extracting more oxygen from the blood as it's delivered to the exercising muscle. Other benefits of cardiovascular training are lowered blood pressure at rest and improvements in your cholesterol.

Strength Training

What happens to a muscle when you lift weights is one of the simplest, yet most misunderstood areas of physiology. Here's the scoop. When you force a muscle to work hard, as in strength training, it increases in size and strength. Simple. This happens by the growth of each individual muscle fiber in a particular muscle. Despite what you may read in some publications, strength training does not increase the number of muscle fibers. In addition, the connective tissue around the muscle increases in strength as well.

Contrary to the myths floating around most gyms (not to mention books and videos), lifting doesn't make a muscle smaller or longer, no matter how many reps you do or what weight you use. Think about it: That guy in the corner of the weight room doing biceps curls isn't doing them to make his arms smaller, yet we often see women doing leg extension or hip exercises in the hopes of "slimming" their thighs. Sorry tummy tuckers, it doesn't work that way. Keep that in mind next time you see someone doing side bends hoping to reduce her waistline.

Stretching

Most people know that they should stretch, but they don't really understand why or what happens when you properly stretch a muscle. Here's a quick rundown.

Stretching allows your muscles to retain elasticity, which prevents injury. With repetitive activities—running, cycling, weight training—certain muscles are used over and over again, which effectively shortens the muscles. This leads to something known as muscular imbalance. When a muscular imbalance occurs, the stronger muscles take over the work of the weaker muscles, causing the weaker muscles to lose so much strength that strains, sprains, and tendinitis occur. For more on this essential ingredient to health and fitness, check out Chapter 7, "Start with Stretching."

Weight Loss

Clearly, losing weight is a frustrating topic for millions of Americans. The good news is that there's a simple formula for weight loss: Eat less and exercise more. Okay, it sounds glib,

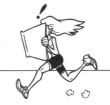

Info to Go

Approximately 18 million Americans are classified as "obese" or at least 30 percent over their ideal body weight.

but it's true. Of course, while it is simple, it's not easy! Nevertheless, the way you lose weight is by burning more calories than you take in. A pound of fat has 3,500 calories worth of energy. That means in order to lose one pound, you need to create a "caloric deficit" of 3,500 calories. The best way to do this is with a combination of decreased caloric intake and increased caloric expenditure.

Here's a nice, neat textbook example. If you decrease your daily intake by 250 calories and increase your activity level enough to burn an extra 250 calories, you'll have a caloric deficit of 500 calories for the day. Multiply that by seven days in a week, and you've got 3,500 calories for the week.

Detraining—Missing Workouts

Now that we've discussed what happens when you work out, let's look at what happens when you don't. (If you're an obsessive-compulsive like Jonathan it means a copious level of angst and guilt.) Surprisingly, many athletes who train often and hard find improved performance after a short layoff. That's due to the fact that many of them are overtrained and in need the rest. Of course, an extended layoff can cause a significant loss in fitness. While there's far less research and information on the topic of detraining than there is on training, there are some basic things to note.

After as little as two weeks of inactivity, there can be measurable decreases in aerobic capacity and muscular strength. This is all the more reason to do all you can to remain active. Remember, just two 30-minute weight-lifting workouts are enough to maintain and even gain strength. Similarly, two or three cardiovascular workouts lasting as little as 15 to 20 minutes can help keep you in shape.

As you read this book, remember that you need to do all you can not to miss workouts. The good news is that we'll help you find the time as well as provide workouts that take less time to maintain or improve your fitness.

The Least You Need to Know

➤ Before embarking on an exercise program, save time and energy by deciding what your needs and goals are.

➤ Working out is not only for looking good, there are numerous health benefits that a consistent fitness program will provide you with.

➤ Muscle size is a function of genetic predisposition; women are not naturally capable of getting muscle-bound by weight training.

➤ If you want to lose weight, eat less, exercise more.

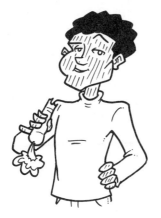

Chapter 4

Nutrition

In This Chapter

➤ Follow the Food Guide Pyramid and do away with fad diets

➤ Restaurants need not be verboten

➤ All servings are not created equal

➤ Have water, will travel

One of the most important aspects of your overall health and fitness is proper nutrition. Eating the right food in the right combination with the right exercise program can pay huge dividends. Unfortunately, a busy lifestyle in a culture littered with fast-food chains can be a major obstacle when you're trying to eat right.

Even if you know what you *should* eat, finding it isn't always easy. Try this one at your local diner: "Waiter, I'd like organic greens with balsamic vinaigrette dressing on the side, four-grain bread, hold the butter, and pasta with marinara sauce." It gets even more challenging at Taco Bell. Factor in grabbing a quick bite at your desk, finding something edible (let alone healthful) on a plane, or whipping something up quickly when you come home from work ravenous, and you've got pepperoni pizza written all over you.

Know Your Nutrients

First, of course, you have to figure out what's healthful. With literally thousands of theories, fad diets, and confusing, even misleading, food labels, that can be a formidable task. Before we talk about specific menu plans and strategies for eating on the go, let's discuss a few basic facts about nutrition.

First, let's take a look at the six essential nutrients. They are …

➤ Carbohydrates   ➤ Vitamins

➤ Protein   ➤ Minerals

➤ Fat   ➤ Water

The first three—carbohydrates (carbs), protein, and fat—supply the calories (energy) for your diet. Carbohydrates can be subdivided into complex or simple. Complex carbs supply sustained energy through a gradual release of glucose into the blood-stream for use as fuel. These are found in pasta, grains, and cereals and should be the mainstays of your training table. Simple carbohydrates—found in soda, jam, cakes, and cookies—are high in sugar and best avoided as a staple of your diet since they tend to cause extreme shifts in blood sugar levels and have little nutritional value.

Protein forms the structural basis of muscle tissue and is used for energy only when there is an insufficient supply of fats and carbohydrates. Meat, poultry, eggs, and legumes are all high-protein foods.

Fats, as you might suspect, are generally chock-full of calories, but low in vitamins and minerals. Certainly, you need some fat in your diet because without it you couldn't process or absorb the fat-soluble vitamins (A, D, E, K).

The next question is how much of each of these nutrients does one need each day? That, dear reader, is the source of considerable debate. However, the smart money according to most nutritionists recommends the following breakdown:

➤ 60 percent to 65 percent of your daily calories should come from carbs.

➤ 10 percent to 12 percent of your daily calories should come from protein.

➤ 20 percent to 30 percent of your daily calories should come from fat.

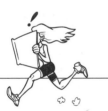

Info to Go

Olive oil, avocados, and nuts, while high in fat, have some nutritional value, unlike other fatty foods such as chips, which have no significant nutrients.

The key to a healthful diet is getting proper amounts of each of these nutrients. When you're armed with the facts and the willingness to plan ahead, it's possible to eat a healthful and tasty diet without driving yourself loco.

First things first. Let's talk about the basics of a healthful diet. After that, we can discuss how to work those guidelines into your lifestyle.

General Nutrition Guidelines

Growing up, most of us heard about the "food groups" and the importance of eating from each of them in order to ensure a safe and healthful diet. A little meat loaf, canned peas, Wonder Bread, and mashed potatoes and you were ready to take on the world—or so they said. In 1992, the U.S. Food and Drug Administration and the U.S. Department of Health and Human Services expanded those four groups to six and represented them in the "Food Guide Pyramid." The Food Guide Pyramid gives a graphic representation of how much we should eat from each of the six categories. They include ...

1. Breads, cereal, pasta, and rice.

2. Vegetables.

3. Fruits.

4. Milk, yogurt, and cheese.

5. Meat, poultry, fish, dry beans, eggs, and nuts.

6. Fats, oils, and sweets.

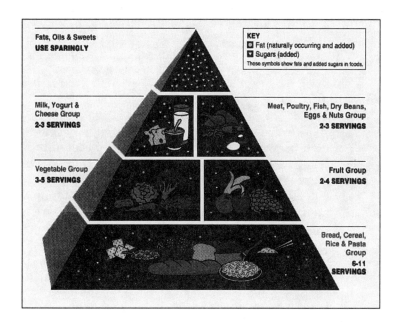

The Food Pyramid gives a good picture of a healthy diet.

Here's the skinny on each of these groups. Obviously, there's volumes written on the subject, but what we really want you to know is the difference between nutritious, "essential" food, and food that doesn't help you achieve optimal health and fitness. Having experienced the gamut of the food spectrum—from Mickey D's to an organic, veggie-based diet—we know of which we speak.

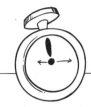

Short Cuts

In the bread, cereal, rice, and pasta food group, a serving is about 32 strands of spaghetti, one slice of bread, half a cup of rice, or one cup of cereal.

A serving of fruit could be an apple, banana, or orange, a wedge of melon, or half a cup of chopped fruit or berries.

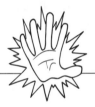

Stop Short

Avoid fruit processed with heavy syrups and juice that is sugar-sweetened. It's also best, whenever possible, to eat organic fruit since it's treated with fewer chemicals and pesticides.

Consuming Your Carbohydrates

As we said, this should be the staple of your diet (roughly 6 to 11 servings per day). The key here is to choose whole-grain products. These are higher in fiber and other nutrients such as vitamins A, B, C, D, B_6, B_{12}, calcium, iron, thiamin, riboflavin, niacin, folic acid, phosphorus, magnesium, zinc, and copper. For example, whole-wheat or seven-grain bread is better than enriched white flour. Brown rice is preferable to white rice. In other words, any product that's been processed is inferior to its more natural brethren.

The other thing to think about is that carbohydrates, or "starchy" foods, aren't fattening if you don't eat them with butter, cheese, or cream sauces. When some people hear that eating a plain bagel with cream cheese isn't the best food choice, they react as if you've told them they're being deported to Rwanda. Making changes to your diet is one of the hardest, most personal, and even most political decisions a person can make. It's also an emotional subject. But if you want to see results and improve the way you look and feel it's worth considering the options.

It's the Berries

While we're sure there are people who don't like fruit, most people salivate when they lay their eyes on an assortment of beautifully displayed fresh fruit. Part of the reason, no doubt, is the taste. Fruit is delicious. But because fruits are such rich sources of vitamins (most notably vitamin C), your body has an inherent craving for these juicy treats.

Try to get at least three servings of fruit per day. If you can, drink fresh fruit juice, at least $3/4$ cup.

Eat Your Veggies

Perhaps because many of us were badgered as kids (dare I say tortured?) by our parents to eat odious green stuff like lima beans, cauliflower, and spinach, vegetables are seen by many people as a chore to eat. That's too bad, since vegetables are high in fiber, low in fat, and filled with vitamins (especially A and C). Vegetables with dark, leafy greens pack the most nutrients per serving. (When in doubt go for kale over beets, broccoli over carrots or corn.)

Again, stay away from lots of butter and salad dressings with sugar and/or hydrogenated vegetable oils. (Hydrogenated fats, like margarine and shortening, can contribute to heart disease.) Eating three to five servings per day is optimal. And going organic is best.

Protein and Its Alternatives

This category gets people hot and bothered. Some claim that eating animal products is bad nutrition as well as bad politics. Everyone must make his or her own decision; however, from a nutritional standpoint, animal products are premium sources of protein, iron, zinc, and B vitamins. Since most of you won't be hunting your own meat sometime soon, it's worth noting that nonorganic beef and poultry contain steroids that many experts say are dangerous to ingest on a regular basis.

Certainly, no such debate exists when you talk about beans, nuts, seeds, and tofu (made from soybeans), which are also excellent sources of protein and other essential nutrients. Nuts make an excellent between-meal snack. Some, like almonds, are fine sources of vitamin E. Try and eat two to three servings from this food group per day.

Devouring Dairy Products

Dairy products are high in calcium and also provide protein and vitamin B_{12}. Here again, there's a healthy debate in the nutrition field on how much of the stuff to knock back. Some experts say that dairy is best avoided, especially people who are "lactose intolerant" (people whose bodies don't digest milk products well). Others say you should try and eat two to four servings per day.

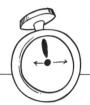

Short Cuts

One serving of vegetables would be one cup of raw leafy greens, half a cup of other chopped vegetables, or $3/4$ cup of vegetable juice.

A serving of protein would include two to three ounces of lean meat, poultry, or fish; one egg, half a cup of beans, and/or two tablespoons of seeds and nuts.

One serving of dairy products equals one cup of milk or yogurt or 1.5 ounces of cheese.

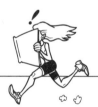

Info to Go

When people are asked to pour a "serving" of cereal, they pour four ounces, while the label serving size *is one* ounce.

For whatever it's worth, Joe stopped eating dairy products a while back and noticed, without changing anything else, he lost body fat and had a bit more bounce in his step. The key is to make sure you're getting enough calcium in your diet (to ensure this, make sure you are getting enough leafy green veggies, which are a rich source of calcium). If you are a big dairy fan, try and choose low-fat products that keep the calories, cholesterol, and saturated fat at a minimum, while keeping all the calcium.

Yum, Yum

This is the category that falls under the "use sparingly" heading. Foods such as fats (all chips, peanut butter, butter, french fries), oils (frying oils), and sweets are the most overused foods in the American diet. Unfortunately for many people, they offer loads of calories but little else nutritionally. (Scooter Pies, anyone?) Two exceptions are vegetable oil (olive oil, flaxseed oil), which is a good source of vitamin E (one tablespoon is enough), and molasses, which is a fine source of iron.

Servings on the Road

When we discussed the six food groups, we gave you an idea of what exactly constitutes a serving. But how do you know how much is enough if you go out to eat?

A good, though less-than-poetic guide to help you figure out what's up, is *Picture Perfect Weight Loss: The Visual Program for Permanent Weight Loss*, by Dr. Howard Shapiro (Rodale). Dr. Shapiro uses common, albeit less-than-savory, examples to give an approximate idea of what a serving size is.

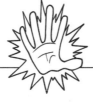

Stop Short

Restaurant portions are usually two to four times larger than a Food Guide Pyramid serving. This usually leads to overeating. (How often have you left a restaurant and uttered this classic phrase: "I'm stuffed!") Food labels usually express serving sizes in ounces, but unless you're walking around with a food scale in your pocket, you're out of luck. At your typical steak house, a portion of meat or poultry is 8 to 12 ounces as opposed to the 2 to 3 ounces outlined in the Food Guide Pyramid.

For example, he says one serving of fruit or vegetables is roughly the size of a tennis ball. A serving of pasta, rice, or cereal? Think hockey puck. A cassette tape is a bread serving and a succulent bar of soap is roughly the size of a serving of meat, poultry, or fish.

When we prepare food at home, there's a tendency to make far more than what's considered a serving. Part of it is practical—leftovers, especially late at night, are more valuable than gold. Part of it is that endurance athletes like Jonathan and Joe, guys whose metabolisms are as high as the Bolivian national debt, eat a lot. At restaurants, as we said, it's worse. Obviously, food should be both enriching and enjoyable. However, what you eat is hugely important and we are the most obese nation in the Western world. Yes, enjoy your food, but it's highly practical to have a few strategies when you eat out so that you don't look down one day and see that you've tacked on 5 or 10 unwanted pounds. With a little thought, you can manage to eat well and still enjoy yourself. Here are some do's and don'ts for dining out.

Dining Out

Do	Don't
When you arrive	
Start with little bread or breadsticks.	Butter them.
Appetizer	
Order a salad with low-fat dressing, or preferably just some lemon juice; olive oil and vinegar is also a good choice.	Order fatty dressings like French, Russian, or blue cheese.
Try raw or stir-fried vegetables.	Order fried and/or breaded appetizers.
Soup	
Choose clear broths, vegetable or noodle soups.	Order cream-of-anything soup.
Entrée	
Go with steamed, baked, or roasted poultry and remove the skin.	Choose anything with the following words: fried, buttered, creamed, au gratin, béarnaise, au lait, crispy, à la mode, *au fromage, buerre blanc,* double-crust, sautéed, panfried, deep-fried, escalloped, *en croûte,* gravy, hollandaise, and prime.
Look for broiled, boiled, poached, baked, and roasted.	

continues

Dining Out   (continued)

Do	Don't
Dessert	
Give fruit or sherbet a try.	Order a skimpy dinner and then eat rich, calorie-filled deserts from everyone else's plate. This is called the Deidre Dinner Special.
Opt for angel food cake if you want something a little more substantial. (Angel food cake will make you feel more virtuous.)	

Here are some tips for specific types of restaurants.

Eating Out at Theme Restaurants

Yes	No
Fast Food	
Grilled chicken sandwiches (no mayo)	Fried chicken
Baked potato (hold the sour cream and butter)	Fried fish
Salads	French fries, burgers
Mexican	
Gazpacho	Refried beans
Rice	Guacamole
Black beans	Nachos
Red beans	Sour cream
Fajitas	
Salsa	
Italian	
Pasta with marinara sauce	Alfredo sauce
Bread	Butter
Salad with vinegar or lemon juice	
Minestrone soup	
Pasta primavera	

Yes	No
Chinese	
Steamed rice	Fried rice
Steamed vegetables	Deep-fried foods
Stir-fried shrimp or chicken	General Tso's chicken
Wonton soup	
Hot-and-sour soup	
Japanese	
Teriyaki	Tempura
Miso soup	
Sushi	
Sashimi	

Another source of extra, unnecessary calories is drinks—both alcoholic and nonalcoholic. Stick with water or sparkling water over colas or other sodas, beer, or other alcoholic beverages. If you're going to drink booze, be restrained. Your pocketbook and body will thank you. We'll talk more about water later, but you can't drink enough.

Also don't be shy about making special requests to your server. When we're out we often ask that our food be prepared in a special way. Our most common request is switching the fries for a baked potato. Hold the butter. Broil the fish or chicken instead of frying it. Often these simple requests make it easy to turn a not-so-nutritious meal into a healthful one.

What if you don't have time to sit down for a real meal and just need to grab a bite at your desk? Snacking between meals is fine; in fact, it often helps prevent you from getting too hungry between meals. No matter how disciplined we are, when our stomachs are grumbling we all have a tendency to eat too much of anything. The trick is finding

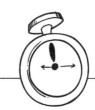

Short Cuts

Try ordering an appetizer as your entrée. Often the food is the same, but the portion is more reasonable—another benefit is that you'll save money.

something healthful. Most of the options at your friendly neighborhood vending machine are far from perfect. Candy bars, chips, and other unhealthful options abound. Even more vexing, lots of foods and snacks that appear fine at first glance are actually foods to stay away from.

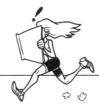

Info to Go

Foods labeled low fat or dietetic aren't always good choices. Just because some of the fat is gone doesn't mean the calories are. Often the decreased fat is simply replaced by extra sugar. (For the record: We prefer original Fig Newtons to the no-fat ones as a healthful snack.)

Here are some common snacks to watch out for:

➤ **Soda.** Undoubtedly this is one of the most common nutritional blunders people make. Countless times we hear, "I watch what I eat but I can't lose weight." On more careful examination, we learn that they down four to five cans of soda a day. Because of the sugar in it, regular soda has about 150 to 200 calories per 12-ounce can. If you drink three cans a day, which is the amount contained in many of the large refillable cups sold by stores and restaurants, you've used up a good share of your recommended daily intake of calories. Water, club soda, or seltzer is a far better alternative. Sugar-free soda is the smarter strategy for weight loss, though it's void of any nutritional value.

➤ **Nuts.** Although they're a good source of protein and vitamin E, just a small handful of nuts can easily contain 100 to 200 calories. For example, there are about 160 calories and 14 grams of fat in those packages of peanuts handed out on airplanes. And just one ounce of sunflower seeds sprinkled on your salad adds 170 calories and about 15 grams of fat.

➤ **Yogurt.** We like yogurt as a snack, but watch out: Not all yogurts are created equal. Many yogurts, including frozen yogurt, may be low in fat but high in sugar and calories. Check the label to see how many calories you're getting. Read labels; just because you read "all natural" on the container, doesn't mean it's the best product on the shelf.

➤ **Muffins.** They seem like a healthful food (especially bran muffins) and they're often sold in so-called health food stores. But one large muffin can have between 300 and 500 calories, not to mention an ample number of fat grams. Don't be fooled by ones labeled "low fat"—they can still be full of calories. Even a regular-size muffin can have 120 to 200 calories. An English muffin or bagel is a better alternative. Low-fat cream cheese or tofu "cream cheese" is better than the real stuff.

➤ **Granola bars.** Oftentimes marketed as "health food," many granola bars are full of simple sugar and fat. Try some fig bars instead.

➤ **Fruit juice.** Certainly better than soda, but still, an eight-ounce serving of orange juice can have 100 to 120 calories, even though an orange has only about 60 calories. Once again, water is a better alternative, or try a piece of fruit. A good alternative is to dilute your juice with water. You get the orange taste without all the calories.

Here are some healthful alternatives when snack time hits:

➤ **Rice cakes** (flavored ones don't taste like Styrofoam).

➤ **Cereal bars** (watch the sugar).

➤ **Pretzels.**

➤ **Breadsticks.**

➤ **Popcorn** (hold the butter).

➤ **Fruit.**

➤ **Crackers** (for example, salt-free saltines).

➤ **Fig bars.**

➤ **Power Bars, Clif Bars,** or one of the many **energy bars** on the market.

As you can see, a little attention to your food choices when you're on the run can make the difference between a healthful diet and one full of nothing but lots of empty calories.

Short Cuts

A light snack between breakfast and lunch is a good way to avoid overeating at lunch. By having a moderately sized lunch with a combination of carbohydrates and protein you can avoid an insulin rush that causes that after-lunch energy drain.

V Is for Vitamins

In the best of all nutritional worlds, you'll get all your vitamins and minerals from your well-balanced, nutrient-dense diet. In reality, there are times when this isn't possible. As a result, it's a good idea for people to take vitamin and mineral supplements in order to round out their diet.

For most people who eat a good, well-rounded diet, vitamin and mineral supplements are unnecessary. However, how many of us do that? While it's unusual to see dangerous vitamin deficiencies, we like to take a multivitamin as a safety net against any missing vitamins or minerals. Outrageous claims made by supplement retailers are quite often full of hyperbole and misinformation and are made in an effort to sell unneeded products. Megadoses of vitamins can be wasteful and in some cases dangerous. So stick with a simple multi and you should be fine.

Supplementation is also important if your diet lacks certain types of food. Vegetarians are often deficient in B_{12}, iron, and zinc, each of which a multivitamin can make up for. In addition, if you have food allergies as Jonathan does—he can't eat most fruits and vegetables—it's a good idea to supplement your vitamin C, because it's impossible to get all your nutrients from your diet.

Water, Water Everywhere

We've saved it for last, but an often overlooked, but absolutely vital part of healthful nutrition, is water. You've probably heard it all before, but the more you hear it the better. Since a male's body is compromised of 60 percent to 65 percent water (women are 50 percent to 60 percent), we need to remain hydrated to function on all cylinders. Also, adequate hydration is crucial to weight loss.

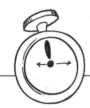

Short Cuts

Keep a pitcher or bottle of water at your desk and take a few sips every 15 minutes or so in order to maintain proper hydration. Remember, don't wait until you're thirsty to drink.

Even people who know the importance of drinking enough water are often underhydrated. Often we hear, "Drinking water is boring." Or, "If I drink eight glasses a day I end up spending half the day in the bathroom." Both are valid comments, but our response is, "Tough!" Why? The downside is too low and the upside too high. Not only does your body process the nutrients it needs when it's properly hydrated, it will help your complexion and overall sense of well-being—a small price to pay compared to a few extra trips to the bathroom.

The Least You Need to Know

➤ By following the Food Guide Pyramid, you can be assured of a healthful diet that will provide you with all of your nutrients without depriving yourself.

➤ Eating in a healthful way doesn't mean you can never eat out. Know what foods to stay away from and take the stress out of restaurant dining.

➤ When you understand what a true serving is, you never have to worry about overindulging.

➤ Water is one of the most important food choices you can ever make—it's the one thing you can never get too much of.

Part 2

The Components of Fitness

This part gives a thorough explanation of each of the major components of fitness: cardiovascular endurance, strength, and flexibility. We show you how to reap the many benefits of cardiovascular training in far less time than you might imagine. We examine basic principles of strength training and look at flexibility, an equally important but often overlooked aspect of fitness. We'll provide strategies for new moms (and dads) who are struggling to regain their shape and balance their child-care and fitness needs.

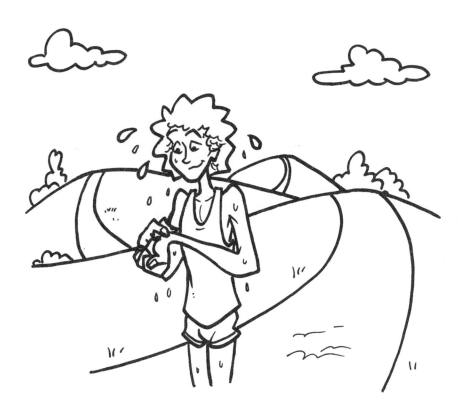

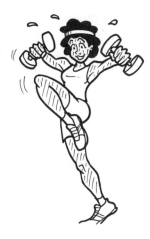

Chapter 5

Aerobics

In This Chapter

➤ Figuring it all out

➤ Target heart rates keep you going

➤ Spinning it out

➤ Stepping it up

We know gym rats with sculpted physiques who regularly drink martinis, smoke, and eat a so-so diet. Many of these guys and gals couldn't run up three flights of stairs without keeling over—despite the fact that they look like extras on *Baywatch.* But are they fit?

Conversely, we know runners and cyclists who crank along religiously but who lack the upper-body strength to bench-press their French poodle let alone their weight. Are they fit?

Fitness is many things to many people. To us, you're as fit as the weakest link in your fitness chain. One of the most neglected areas of fitness in our muscle-obsessed culture is cardiovascular conditioning.

Your Cardiovascular System

There are many benefits to strengthening your *cardiovascular (CV) system,* including weight and body fat loss, improved blood cholesterol level, decreased blood pressure, and decreased risk for diabetes and other serious conditions. Combine strength training and stretching with cardiovascular (cardio, or aerobic) training and you have a formula for fitness.

Many people, especially us urban gym rats, get stuck in a rut and begin to dread aerobic exercise. That's because we lack the creativity or courage to try something else and end up plugging away on the treadmill or StairMaster like an assembly line worker at the factory. While our aim is to help you find the time to work out, laboriously slogging through your cardio routine is unnecessary. That's because there are countless ways to skin that cardio cat.

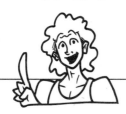

Workout Words

Your **cardiovascular (CV) system** consists of the heart, lungs, and blood vessels that deliver blood from the heart to the muscles and then back to the lungs.

Outdoors in the "real world" you can walk, run, ride a bike, in-line skate, cross-country ski, canoe, swim, even chase squirrels. Indoors, you've got treadmills, cross-country ski simulators, rowing ergometers, elliptical trainers, stair climbers, a variety of bikes, and even climbing walls in some of the trendier gyms out there. (Don't get us started on the variety of aerobic resources available.) And when in doubt, there's always that staircase waiting to be ascended. With all these options—and we urge you to try as many as possible—you're sure to have something that will keep the boredom at bay.

Define Your CV Goals

We humans are rather quirky and complex beings. One side of our brain seeks comfort and pleasure. Our couch potato side likes nothing better than lounging on satin cushions as we're hand-fed succulent grapes. Another side of us craves discipline and enjoys setting goals—to make more money, travel to Tibet, to get in great shape. Without goals, it seems, we tend to flounder without making much progress from thought to reality.

In most ways, it doesn't matter what your motivation is, as long as it helps get you going. Whether you want to shape up to go to your twentieth high school reunion or try out for the Toledo Mud Hens, your goal becomes a road map—a guide to keep you on track to your destination. Without this personal pull the only place you're likely to wind up is right where you started.

Often simply telling people about the benefits of having a fitness goal isn't enough. During Jonathan's first meeting with a client, he explained cardiovascular training—stuff like weight loss, improved sports performance, fat loss, and increased muscular definition, as well as decreased risk of high blood pressure, diabetes, and other serious medical conditions. His client, a stout middle-aged businessman, looked at him vacantly. "Yeah, yeah," he said impatiently, "but I want to beat Snodgrass at the Corporate Challenge next month." (The Corporate Challenge is a series of 3.5-mile running races held in Central Park each summer.) Ironically (or not), edging that smug Mr. Snodgrass at the finish line provided ample motivation for him to follow Jonathan's plan.

The three most frequently asked questions we hear in this realm are ...

1. How often do I have to do my cardio exercise?
2. What's the best cardiovascular exercise?
3. How long do I have to do it?

Ready for this definitive answer? It depends!

If your primary goal is to live a long, healthy life but you couldn't give a hoot about improving your 5K time—let alone run a marathon—take a look at the recommendations made by the American College of Sports Medicine (ACSM), which lists the minimum requirements necessary for the enhancement of health and cardiorespiratory fitness.

ACSM Minimum Requirements

The American College of Sports Medicine lists four categories you should know about:

➤ **Mode of aerobic activity.** This is defined as any activity that uses large muscle groups that can be maintained for a prolonged period of time, for example, running-jogging, walking-hiking, swimming, skating, bicycling, rowing, cross-country skiing, rope skipping, and more.

➤ **Intensity of exercise.** This is defined as physical activity corresponding to 55 percent to 90 percent of your maximum heart rate.

➤ **Duration of exercise.** This category includes a wide range, anywhere from 15 to 60 minutes of continuous (or discontinuous) aerobic activity.

➤ **Frequency of exercise.** From three to five days a week.

There are two things to take note of here. First, don't think you can plug away at the minimum recommendations and be ready to ride in the Tour de France. It will, however, help transform someone in poor shape, as well as help someone who already works out maintain a decent level of fitness and health.

The second important point is the phrase "continuous or discontinuous aerobic activity." That means that walking up the stairs or power walking half a mile to the railroad instead of hopping in the car counts toward the total. Again, for a busy professional, using your time efficiently—which often means finding creative ways to work out—can mean the difference between being fit or being fat.

Your Target Heart Rate

Again, the goal aspect of training comes into play. If you're hoping for a little more than just overall health, it's a good idea to factor in some more direction and precision. Enter the *target heart rate.* Armed with this simple fact, you'll ensure that you are exercising at the proper intensity. Why bother? First, most people who do regular cardio work simply don't go hard enough. We routinely see people at the gym reading *The New York Times* from cover to cover without breaking a sweat. (Joe even knows one guy who drinks coffee while he rides the stationary bike, reads, and listens to music on his Walkman. Basically, the man is moving his legs in circles in an ersatz coffee shop.) And there are a select (albeit smaller) group of people who get on the treadmill and run like lemmings sprinting off a cliff. (This is a classic prescription for injury and frustration.) It's very useful in this early stage of building cardio fitness to figure out what your target heart rate is.

There are two formulas that you can use to figure it out. The first formula starts by figuring out your maximum heart rate (MHR):

1. Calculate your predicted maximum heart rate: 220 minus your age.

2. Take that figure and multiply it by 60 percent. This represents the low end of your target heart rate.

3. Multiply your predicted maximum heart rate by 85 percent. This is the high end of your target heart rate.

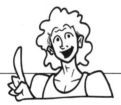

Workout Words

Target heart rate (THR) is the most efficient zone within which you gain a significant cardiovascular benefit from your aerobic exercise. Exercising below your THR will not produce much in the way of cardiovascular gains (though you will still burn some calories), while most people will find that exceeding their THR will be very painful and hard to maintain for more than a couple of minutes.

For example:

Deidre is 37 years old, so her predicted maximum heart rate is $220 - 37 = 183$

The low end of her target zone is $183 \times 60\% = 110$

The high end of her target is $183 \times 85\% = 156$

The second, more accurate way to figure your target heart rate during aerobic activity is called the Karvonen, or heart rate reserve method formula. First you need to record your resting heart rate (RHR). To get an accurate reading, take your pulse first thing in the morning before you get out of bed on three consecutive days. Average the three, and take that to be your resting heart rate (RHR). Here's the rest of the equation:

1. 220 minus your age is your predicted maximum heart rate (MHR).

2. MHR minus your resting heart rate (RHR).

3. Multiply that number by 60 percent and 85 percent.

4. Add your RHR to each of these values for the low end and high end of your target heart rate zone.

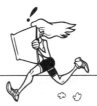

Info to Go

The formula for predicting maximum heart rate (220 minus your age) is a rough estimate and can vary greatly among individuals. Consequently, some people may need to adjust their training zone according to their true maximum heart rate. Physiologists can determine your maximum heart rate in a lab setting.

This may sound complicated but it's really not. Let's figure it out for the 37-year-old Deidre, who has a resting heart rate of 72.

Here's how she would figure out her target heart rate:

$$220 - 37 = 183$$
$$183 - 72 = 111$$
$$111 \times .60 = 66.2$$
$$72 + 66.2 = \mathbf{138.2}$$

Once you know what your target heart rate is, you can monitor your pulse while you are exercising to ensure that you are working out at the correct intensity depending on your goal that day. The low end of the zone is at the "easiest" you should work out if you want to get significant improvements in your cardiovascular system.

You want to be at 60 percent to 65 percent when you're doing longer cardio workouts. The high end of the target heart rate provides the greatest cardiovascular benefit, but will also be very hard for most people to maintain for any length of time. Physiologically, the longer you work out, the more efficient you'll become—meaning you'll go faster at the same level of exertion.

How Long Is a Heartbeat?

There are two places you can use to take your pulse: your radial pulse, which is on the thumb side of your wrist, or your carotid pulse, which is located on your neck on

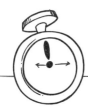

Short Cuts

If you take your pulse at your carotid artery, be sure not to press too hard. Just a light touch is all it takes. Too much pressure on the artery can result in a sudden decrease in blood pressure and cause you to black out in the middle of a workout.

either side of your throat. Use your index and middle finger to check your pulse at either site. When you are ready to take the pulse, the very first count is zero, then one, then two, then three, and so on, until you've reached 10 seconds. Take the number and multiply by six.

If all this seems too complicated or too much like work, go out and buy a wireless heart rate monitor. Polar is the best known and most popular brand, though Cardiosport and others are becoming increasingly popular. These handy devices consist of a chest strap/transmitter that sends a signal to a digital watch, which measures your heart rate with EKG-like precision. In addition, monitors with stopwatches and beepers that tell you when you're above or below your training zone are available.

Wireless heart rate monitors are simple to use and as accurate as an EKG.

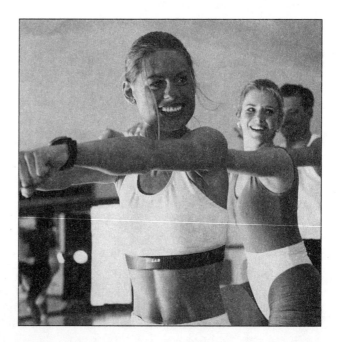

Eating Before Workouts

We discussed general nutrition principles in Chapter 4, "Nutrition"; let's now talk about a few things to keep in mind about eating before heading out for your cardio workout.

Depending on whom you ask, the only thing worse than working out on an empty stomach is working out when you're full. In the former instance, you're likely to hit the wall and pay the piper when your blood sugar level drops and your energy level follows. Exercising with a full gut can cause all sorts of gastrointestinal discomfort and grind your workout to a halt.

Jonathan can wolf down a pound of spaghetti and happily go for a spin on his bike an hour later. On the other hand, Deidre would be on her hands and knees if she followed the same plan. For her, and most others, a piece of fruit or a bagel an hour before a workout is enough to finish the workout without providing any stomach agitation.

Also make sure you're well hydrated before you hit the cardio trail. Waiting until you're thirsty to start drinking is too late. The key here is making sure your urine is clear. (Although taking vitamins will throw you off here.) If it's not, you need to drink more.

Choosing Your CV Machine

Here's an amusing fact. If you read the promotional literature from treadmill retailers, stationary bikes, cross-country ski machines, and rowers and you'll see that they all claim to be the best mode of aerobic activity on the market. Obviously, most of those "studies" are biased toward a particular product. In fact many of them are performed or paid for by the equipment company and are as impartial as a hanging judge.

The question remains: Which machines are best? Each has its merits, both theoretical and practical. In fact, the best machine is the one you'll use. Let's take a well-designed, state-of-the-art machine that you consider only slightly more attractive than a medieval torture device. Odds are that you're not going to use it ever, let alone consistently. For this reason and more, it's best to jump from one piece of equipment as regularly as a teenager changes outfits. (This can be done from workout to workout or even within the same session.) On those days when you're feeling frisky and have extra time, you could row for 20 minutes on the Concept II erg and tack on another 20 minutes on the Versaclimber. This also saves you from the faux pas of exceeding the time limit on the equipment and risking the ire of your gym mates.

Stop Short

Unless you're enamored with one particular machine—give me the treadmill or give me death—or you're training for a competitive event and need, say, to ride your favorite exercise bike for fear or turning into a toad, there's no reason to use the same machine every day. Not only will the variety help you avoid overuse injuries, this ensures that you work a variety of muscles.

Classy Exercise

Unless you're working out in a pure "muscle-head" gym that feature little more than free weights and machines, most gyms offer a variety of classes. These are great because most are well structured and pack a lot of heart-thumping activity into a short amount of time. Also, even if you're feeling blasé, all you have to do is show up and the teacher will get you going.

The big question is which class do you take? Like restaurants in Manhattan, there are scores of them and each has its own special flavor. Here's a quick guide to what kind of classes you can expect to find in the fitness world.

Spin, Baby, Spin

Spin classes are the hottest ticket in town these days and if you like group settings, hot music, and bicycles this is just what the cycling doctor ordered. "Spinning" was invented in the mid-1990s by a West Coast bicycle racer who goes by the name of Johnny G.

We've taken a host of spin classes taught by a variety of teachers. Some, usually led by aerobics teachers, are very festive, almost stationary dances to raucous music. (Add a bar and a cocktail waitress and you'd swear you were at a club on a Saturday night.) Others, usually taught by cyclists, are more streamlined, with the hard-core cyclist in mind. Kirk Whiteman, former world champion cyclist, teaches one of the best spinning classes around. Mr. Whiteman, a muscular 34-year-old with quads as hard as a grand piano, gives the following suggestions for finding a good spinning class:

➤ Make sure there is an adequate warm-up period.

➤ Make sure that the instructor reviews all bicycle safety procedures, such as how to stop as well as how to properly affix the toe clips.

➤ Make sure the instructor corrects poor posture or incorrect positioning.

➤ Make sure there is an adequate cool-down period.

➤ Check to make sure that your instructor is certified as a group cycling teacher. Improper bike setup is a guaranteed way to hurt your knees.

To some, stepping into this world of spinning madness can be intimidating. Fret not. After the first class you'll feel right at home. The key when you're starting out is not to attempt anything that you feel uncomfortable with. Many instructors will have you stand up out of the "saddle" or stand up and sit down as part of the routine. This is fine, but be careful not to plop down onto the seat. Over time, you're likely to suffer from lower back pain and may need to head to a physical therapist.

Step It Up

Step aerobics hit the scene in the early '90s. These classes have you hop up and down on a step to get your heart rate up. There are different step heights to choose from—the higher the step, the more intense the exercise.

One of the temptations when you first take one of these classes is to try to keep up with more experienced class members. Resist that urge and go at your own pace. The first time Joe, a nationally ranked marathon kayaker, jumped into one of these classes, he followed the 50-year-old woman in front of him, and needed medical assistance to get out of bed the next morning. If you find that the pace of the class is just too fast, don't stop—stopping will cause blood to pool in your legs—just slow down or alter you movement. For example, if the instructor wants you to jump but your legs are thrashed, instead hop from side to side at a comfortable pace.

Again, we can't stress the importance of proper hydration. Hopping around in a small room with 20 other jumping jacks is a sweaty affair. Drink 8 to 16 ounces of water 30 to 60 minutes before exercise, 4 to 10 ounces of water every 15 minutes during your workout, and another 8 to 16 ounces after exercise.

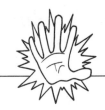

Stop Short

Since most aerobics classes, with the exception of spinning, require side-to-side movement, the possibility of spraining your ankle exists. When buying sneakers, make sure they are built to support you in lateral movements.

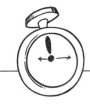

Short Cuts

Many of the early aerobic dance tapes and classes contained countless movements that were actually bad for you. So make sure to look for classes and tapes taught by certified instructors, not dancers.

Aerobics Class

The oldie but goodie, aerobic dance classes are still a mainstay in health clubs and home exercise tapes. Ranging from high impact (lots of jumping) to low impact (no jumping), a good aerobic dance class is a fun way to work your upper and lower body as well as add to your repertoire of moves you can use on the dance floor. Like spin and step classes, the instructor tries to motivate you to push a little harder than you can push yourself. Don't confuse this with marine boot camp. A good teacher will make sure that you're working at a pace comfortable for you.

In the end, the most important thing is, first, to make sure that you do some form of aerobic activity. Second, do something you enjoy. And third, try and stay within your target zone for workouts of more than a few minutes.

The Least You Need to Know

➤ Define your goals to stay on track.

➤ Eating properly before you exercise will keep you from hitting the wall in the middle of your workout.

➤ Mixing up your exercise routine will keep you from being bored.

➤ If you need company to motivate you to work out, classes are a good way to go.

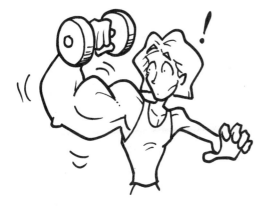

Chapter 6

Strengthening

In This Chapter

➤ Why strengthen?

➤ Grow strong in your golden years

➤ Getting down to basics

➤ Home is where the equipment is

Considering that we are also the authors of *The Complete Idiot's Guide to Weight Training,* you can bet the family fortune that the three of us are staunch advocates of strength training. Here's why. One of the neat things about strength training is that it can have countless benefits for everyone—from teens to the elderly, male, female, large and small. Want to look, good? Lift. Prevent injury? Lift. Boost your metabolism and lose fat? Improve your game? Feel better? Lift, lift, and lift. (Did we say lift?)

Again, we often hear the familiar refrain, "Okay, so weight training is great, but I don't have the time." Here's the thing that surprises most people. If you know what you're doing, making significant gains from lifting takes far less time than you think. Many lifting aficionados like to lift for an hour (or more) a day, three or four times a week, dividing their body by muscle groups. Typically they work different muscles each day and usually take three- to four-minute rests between sets. That's fine and dandy, but horribly inefficient.

In this chapter we'll discuss the benefits and basic principles of strength training and show you why it takes far less time than you may think to help you meet your fitness goals.

The Strength Debate

When people think about strength training, usually all they think of are bigger, more defined-looking muscles. Fortunately there's a lot more to it than that. Sure, muscles look good, but they serve lots of other purposes too. Before we discuss the basic principles of strength training, let's take a look at the benefits.

Muscle Turns Heads

While we'll give you plenty of practical reasons why you should lift weights, for most people building bone density and preventing debilitation in the golden years isn't their main motivation. Let's face it, muscle is attractive. If you doubt it, go to Florence and visit Michelangelo's towering nude sculpture of *David*—an awe-inspiring representation of the male ideal. Whether it's six-pack abs, broad shoulders (remember, broad shoulders make your waist and hips look narrower), or toned legs, we all want muscle.

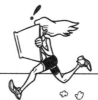

Info to Go

In 1996, when Joe was training to run the hundredth Boston Marathon, he was running along a crowded sidewalk toward Prospect Park in Brooklyn. Walking in the opposite direction was a conservatively dressed matronly woman in her 60s. After Joe jogged by, she turned around and hollered in a sweet Southern accent, "Nice legs, honey!" The big lug kept smiling halfway around the park.

Muscle is preferable to fat for a variety of reasons. First, it's aesthetically more pleasing. Because muscle is denser than fat, a pound of muscle takes up less space (or volume) than a pound of fat. That explains why Deidre, who weighs 130 pounds and has 16 percent body fat, wears size four or six pants and a size four dress. Contrast her with another 130-pounder, Ms. Not So Slim. However, this woman has 25 percent body fat. Because Not So Slim's 130 pounds are made up of more fat and less muscle, she cuts a larger figure than Deidre, and wears a size 8 or 10. In other words, when you add muscle mass the scale may say more, but your wardrobe says less.

Another very potent reason why people who strength train keep at it is that they find they can eat more than they could before they started lifting, add muscle, and look even better.

Faster Metabolisms Burn Calories

Not only does muscle weigh more than fat, muscle is more metabolically active. Huh? Here's the skinny on fat. Even at rest, our bodies burn calories. But because muscle, not fat, burns calories at rest, the more muscle you have, the more calories you burn. The amount of calories that a pound of muscle burns each day is a topic of some debate in the scientific community. Some say it's as much as 50 calories; however, we're not convinced it's more than 20 or so. Regardless, we know that becoming a more efficient calorie-burning machine while you sleep, watch TV, or talk on the phone is added incentive to follow through on a daily workout regime. Remember, the more muscle you have, the higher your metabolism.

Ouch Control

One of the first things athletes in all sports do immediately after surgery is rehab with weights. While it sounds counterintuitive—why work an injured body part—stronger muscles make for greater protection against injury by reducing the stress on joints such as your knees, hips, and shoulders.

While many athletes lift to help improve their performance, we feel that the most important reason to lift is injury prevention. Jonathan lifts year-round, not only to help his cycling, but also to help him avoid the back, neck, and knee injuries that are common among cyclists. Less injury means more saddle time, which means better performance. This, in turn, means a healthier, happier Jonathan. Talk about a grand cycling cycle.

Another persuasive reason to strength train is the effect it has on minimizing *osteoporosis*. In her job as a physical therapist, Deidre constantly sees the damaging effects of osteoporosis on senior citizens. Before you get smug on us and skip this section comforted by the thought that you're light-years away from being elderly, you should know that due to physical inactivity and poor diet, signs of osteoporosis, while far more common in older populations are becoming increasingly common among women in their mid- to late 20s!

Here's a quick anatomy lesson. Bones maintain their structure over time through a process of old bone removal (resorption) and new bone formation. In early adulthood, the rates of loss and replacement are balanced. As women age and go through menopause, roughly between the ages of 46 and 54, their estrogen levels drop and the rate of bone removal outpaces the rate of bone replacement. Incredibly, 25 million women are affected by osteoporosis—one out of five women over the age of 45, and 4 out of 10 women over the age of 75.

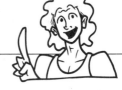

Workout Words

Osteoporosis is a condition where the bones become soft and brittle due to loss of tissue. Women and men afflicted with this are prone to bone breakage, especially of the hip.

You can prevent (or severely retard) this from occurring through weight training. When skeletal bone is subjected to 10 times the amount of strain that is required for typical daily activities, it responds by creating stronger tissue. That is one reason why weight training is so valuable for not only older women but younger ones as well.

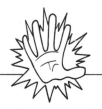

Stop Short

While osteoporosis is thought of almost exclusively as a woman's disease, the fact is that 3.5 million men over the age of 50 suffer from this disease due primarily to decreasing levels of testosterone.

Here's another surprising fact: Women in their 20s can also fall victim to osteoporosis, in large part due to our countries' obsession with dieting. A young woman who limits her intake to 1,200 or 1,300 calories a day by relying heavily on diet soda, rice cakes, and salads is not getting the calcium and vitamin D that her body requires. Look at an x-ray of someone on this anemic diet and you'll see the bones of a 60-year-old osteoporotic woman. Couple this with the stress of vigorous aerobic workouts and you have a body under constant assault without the tools to rebuild itself. Often the result is injury, illness, and depression.

Life 101

While lifting weights will improve your appearance and athletic performance, there's a very practical side to gaining strength. It's called daily living. Though less impressive than towing tractor-trailers or pulling a piano from a burning building, the added strength you gain from weight lifting can help immeasurably with normal, everyday activities.

Anyone who's ever traveled on the New York City subway has seen this scene countless times. One woman with two or three children is schlepping a stroller, groceries, and baby supplies up three steep flights of crowded concrete steps. Negotiating this minefield makes jousting an American Gladiator seem positively serene. While this Herculean feat of strength is born of necessity, it would be far less strenuous if that mom were a regular at the gym.

The same is obviously true whether carrying groceries or moving your sofa. The problem is that once you get real strong, your friends will start asking you to help them move. "You're the only one I know without a bad back," is the comment Joe frequently hears. Of course, you can say that you'd love to help but you're too thrashed from lifting weights and can barely lift a playing card.

Sad But True

The biggest reason the elderly are forced to move from their own homes to assisted-living residences or nursing homes is that they are no longer capable of taking care of themselves. Typically the saga begins when they're no longer able to walk outside alone. Next it becomes a necessity to hire a home aide to do the daily chores of living. Then the ability to get in and out of the bathtub becomes so limited that bathing is often neglected. The last straw is a fall that leaves them unable to get up on their own.

Scary business, but unfortunately true. As we stated earlier, by the age of 60 or 70, you've lost 30 percent to 40 percent of your muscle mass—making everyday activities such as climbing stairs or standing up from a chair especially challenging. Muscle drives the skeleton. Without it, how do you move?

Clearly these are more than a few reasons to underscore the value of strength training. Now let's examine the basic principles behind this stuff.

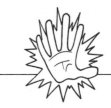

Stop Short

Remember when muscle mass is lost, balance often goes with it. Your muscle is what supports your skeleton. With a decrease in muscle mass, you become weak and your ability to remain steady and stable is compromised.

Principled Strength

Developing a solid and efficient strength-training program that fits your body and schedule isn't rocket science; however, the specifics that govern the best routine(s) for you are based on several basic strength-training principles that should be considered whether you're in the gym, on the road, or at home.

Choice of Exercise

Train all major muscle groups: legs, back, chest, shoulders, arms, and abdominal muscles (abs). Skipping muscles can cause imbalances and lead to injury. Since time is important, skip isolation exercises such as flyes (chest) and lateral raises (shoulders) and focus on compound movements such as leg presses, bench presses, and lateral pull downs that work multiple muscle groups in one exercise. Isolation exercises are fine for bodybuilders who need to train every obscure muscle that's visible in a tiny swimsuit, but not very time-effective for the rest of us.

Progression of Exercise

Work from larger to smaller muscles, such as the muscles of your chest, back, and shoulders before your arms. If you train smaller muscles such as your arms first, they'll be too tired to help you when they're needed for your back, chest, and shoulder exercises.

Frequency

Aim for two to three workouts per week on nonconsecutive days. It's important to remember that muscles need time to recover from strength-training workouts. So while it's ambitious, even noble, to lift five or six days a week, it's also misguided. That's also good news if you don't want to have your calls and mail forwarded to the gym.

Sets

One *set* of lifting, when done properly, is as effective as doing two, three, or more sets. It certainly is far more efficient. There are a lot of scholarly studies on this subject, but trust us on this one. One of our favorite references is the web site www.cyberpump.com.

Reps

Forget all that stuff you've read about high *reps* for "tone" and low weight for "bulk." Ten to twelve reps per set is plenty. The most important variable that determines how your muscle responds to the exercise is how hard you're working on your last rep.

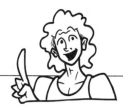

Workout Words

A repetition, or **rep** in gyms-peak, is the execution of an strength-training exercise one time. For instance, one rep of a bench press includes pushing the bar from your chest until your arms are fully extended, followed by returning the bar to your chest. A **set** is a series of repetitions performed consecutively. For example, you might do a set of 10 reps of the bench press.

Weight

Find the resistance that allows you to do no fewer than 10, but not more than 12 reps. When you get strong enough to complete 12 reps, increase the weight by 5 percent or so. Don't lock in on the same amount of reps, workout after workout, or you'll never get stronger. Variety is the spice of life and a key ingredient in improving your fitness.

Speed of Movement

When you're lifting, the ideal is three seconds positive (on the exertion) and three seconds negative (the return). The bad news is that's considerably slower than most people lift. The good news is you'll get much better results and decrease your chance of injury. Men, who are typically more interested in how much weight they lift rather than how well they lift, resist this more. You'll probably find that by slowing down and eliminating momentum, you'll have to lighten your load.

Rest Between Sets

You should rest for one to two minutes between sets. That gives you enough time to move from one exercise to another, recover from the effort, and even work in with a training partner if you've got one. When they actually time the amount of rest they allow between sets, most people discover that they were resting far longer than two minutes.

Remember our consistent refrain: Two or three 30-minute workouts a week won't get you on the cover of *Mega Muscle Man* magazine. They can, however, be enough to improve your strength and fitness dramatically as well as have a major impact on your appearance. The keys to making sure that an efficient strength-training workout is an effective one are choice of exercise and intensity. Choose the wrong exercises, or do a half-hearted job, and you might as well stay home and read *Mega Muscle* instead. Choose your exercises wisely and work hard and you're off to the races.

In Parts 2, 3, and 4 we'll outline specific routines to do given a specific time frame—from a few quick calisthenics in your office to a 20-minute routine you can do on the road to full-body routines here, abroad, or in a dark coat closet. In short, if you've got the will, we've got the routine.

Working Out at Home

The spiel we usually hear from people with more ambition than time is, "That's great, but I can't get to the gym." Once again, sounds good, but we're unmoved. Here's why. There are lots of things you can do to stimulate your muscles without going to a gym. While fitness professionals debate the merits of machines versus free weights, Cybex versus Nautilus, and more, there's a tendency to overestimate the intelligence of your muscles. We're here to tell you that your muscles don't care much if they're pushing against a barbell, a Nautilus weight stack, a rubber band, a pile of two-by-fours, or your stubborn mule.

Yes, there are some theoretical and practical advantages to each method, but our point is that you shouldn't get bogged down in them. That's because there are far more important variables that you can control that affect your workout such as choice of exercises, intensity, and rest between exercises. Even a world champion power lifter such as Deidre has been known to improvise when necessary. On the road, she's used a broomstick (with the 180-pound Jonathan providing the resistance), rubber bands, tubing, and anything else she can lay her calloused hands on.

A sensible solution for those who truly can't get to the gym is traveling the home workout route. Unless you're Donald Trump, it's unlikely that you'll be setting up a home gym comparable to what you can find in a commercial fitness center. Nevertheless, there are some solid options available that won't take up a ton of space or force you to take out a second mortgage.

One option is the multifunction machines that enable you to do a variety of exercises. The three most popular are the Total Gym, SOLOFLEX, and BOWFLEX. Each machine has been around for years and comes with complete assembly and usage instructions.

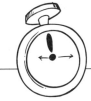

Short Cuts

Each of these machines is capable of handling users of various shapes and sizes and can help both men and women build strong, shapely muscles.

The Total Gym uses your body weight as resistance and is easily stored away.

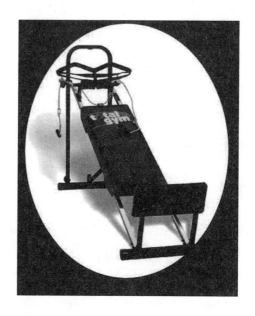

The SOLOFLEX uses rubber bands rather than weights for resistance.

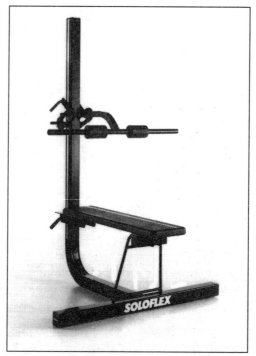

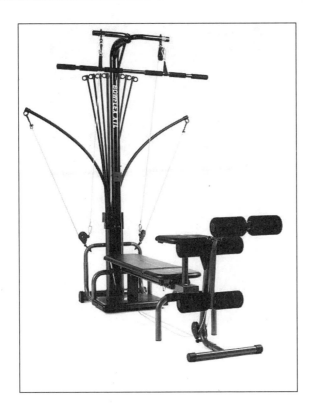

Power Rods create the resistance on the BOWFLEX.

Though all three are well built, reliable, and versatile, of the three, we prefer the BOWFLEX. It has a variety of exercises and is adjustable and solidly designed. Our biggest question is whether you'll ever look like the model that you see in their infomercials. Sure, the Adonis in the ad is lean and mean, but odds are he worked long and hard pumping iron. Regardless, each of these machines can help you get strong and spare you a trip to the gym.

Free Weights

If you don't have the space at home but still can't get to the gym, working out with dumbbells on your on turf is the way to go. An adjustable bench, a barbell, and some dumbbells are enough to allow you to do a variety of strength-training exercises for your entire body. If you're pressed for space (pun intended), we particularly like an adjustable set of dumbbells called the PowerBlock. For about $200, The PowerBlock allows you to adjust the weight of the barbell easily and quickly from 5 to 45 pounds.

In Parts 3 and 4 we'll lay out specific routines to help get you strong in a minimum of time.

PowerBlock is a great space-saving option in place of conventional dumbbells.

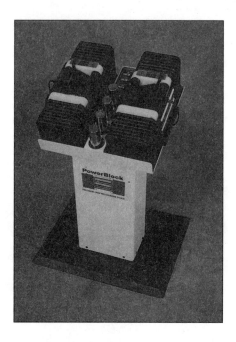

The Least You Need to Know

➤ There are more reasons to strengthen than to look good.

➤ The elderly don't have to be frail and homebound; exercising benefits them, too.

➤ Understanding the basics of exercising can get you better results in less time.

➤ If you don't have time for the gym, you can get a good workout at home.

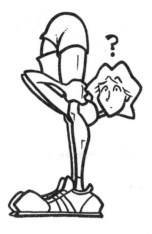

Chapter 7

Start with Stretching

In This Chapter

➤ Why stretching is important

➤ Stretch long and prosper

➤ Stretches for all activities

➤ Yoga and you

So you have less time than you usually do at the gym today. Though you had scheduled some stretching into your workout, your tight schedule (pun intended) means that something has to go. If you're like most people, including us, the first thing to fly out the gym window is stretching, which ironically happens to be one of the most important facets of a fitness regime. If you neglect this vital part of working out, you're far more likely to suffer the nagging injuries that often put nonstretchers on the disabled list.

Why is stretching so crucial? Virtually all repetitive activities shorten our muscles—cycling, running, walking, strength training, you name it. And everyday stuff such as standing, sitting, driving, even lying on the couch watching TV are much the same. (A yoga teacher we know said the best way to get loose is to get rid of our furniture.) However, unless you're going to have a huge yard sale, the only way to counteract all of this "shortening" is by restoring elasticity to your muscles. Stretching, sports fans, is your secret weapon.

All of us are genetically predisposed to a certain degree of flexibility. Just watch an infant suck on his or her toes and you'll realize how naturally bendy kids are. However, no matter how flexible we are in the beginning, as we age our muscles get stiffer, unless, of course, we consciously work at it. While there's no need to emulate the circus contortionist, if your muscles are chronically tight you're an accident waiting to happen. Did you say bad back? Stiff neck? Problems with your sciatic nerve? Keep reading.

Why Me?

Our muscles work best when they are a specific length, which is different for every muscle in your body. When muscles become tight, say from sitting in a slouched position eight hours per day five days per week, very often spasms result because the muscles are working hard to sustain this unnatural posture. Very often physical therapists hear stories from people with strained or torn muscles who say "all" they did was jump up to get the phone and, boom, they pulled something in their hip. That's because they've been sitting all day. And when they hustled to the phone, their severely compromised hip muscles said, "Nope, not today. I'm too tight and sore to jump up like that."

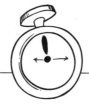

Short Cuts

Always do a light warm-up before stretching, otherwise you risk injuring those cold muscles. That's especially true when working out first thing in the morning. In a perfect world, we prefer warming up on a machine like a cross-country ski machine or a bike that uses both your arms and legs, but anything that will promote a little blood circulation will do fine. A short, brisk walk can fill the bill.

Very often a tight body and a tense mind go hand in hand (or mind and body). That's why one of the best reasons to stretch is that it's a great stress reliever. Sitting peacefully on a mat, consciously breathing into the stretch, is the perfect tonic for us achiever types who feel the need to run around accomplishing stuff all day. Add some soothing music to the mix and you're really cruising. An added benefit is that it's an opportunity to reflect on what's ahead (or behind) you. You can use it as an opportunity to come up with new ideas or just daydream. For some, stretching is a form of meditation.

Stretching is basically a simple and relaxing activity, but there are a few basics that you need to keep in mind.

Stretching 101

Quite often, we see people in the gym stretching all wrong. In an effort to help you unlearn any bad habits you might have picked up over the years, here's a series of tips to keep in mind as you stretch.

➤ **Never bounce.** This is also called ballistic stretching, the old-fashioned touch-your-toes-no-matter-what stretching you did back in high school. This aggressive approach—favored by sadistic gym teachers and snarling drill sergeants—can leave you less flexible than doing nothing. Worse, it can hurt you. The only people who do this today are those who don't know any better.

➤ **Stretch gently.** Stretching isn't like lifting weights where you want to squeeze out one final rep to stimulate maximum muscle growth. In this realm, the point is to stretch only to the point where you feel a gentle sensation in the muscle—never pain. Push too hard and you're doing far more harm than good. In fact, nothing drives us crazier than seeing some well-meaning guy (it's almost always men) on the floor grimacing as he strains to touch his toes that loom off in the distance.

➤ **Hold each stretch for 20 to 30 seconds.** Anything shorter and you probably won't get much benefit. A good way to do this is to hold the stretch for 10 deep breaths. If you're not stretching too far this should feel good.

➤ **Breathe deeply.** Another big no-no in the stretching game is people who act like pearl divers and hold their breath midstretch. As you hold the stretch, breathe deeply, stretching just a little farther with each exhalation. Again, don't push so far so that it's painful.

Sidestep Injury

We mentioned how a sedentary person jumping up to answer the phone can pull a hip muscle. Happens all the time; however, we know countless athletes who experience much the same thing, for different but similar reasons. For example, a cyclist or runner is walking (not running) across the street, steps off the curb, and "pop"—there goes the calf muscle. Odds are—in fact we'd bet our donuts on it—that neither of these athletes stretched regularly (if at all). Their respective recreational activities left them so tight that something as routine as walking across the street pushed them over the edge.

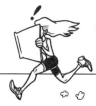

Info to Go

One of the best indicators of back pain and/or potential injury is the *sit-and-reach* test. Sit on the floor with straight legs and bend forward at the waist toward your toes. If your fingertips can't reach your toes, it's a sure sign that you need to work on your hamstring and lower-back flexibility.

While we'll spare you the long-winded lesson in anatomy, trust us that our muscles depend on each other to be both symmetrical and loose. If your hamstrings are tight, your back is often sounding an alarm; if your shoulders are too tight, your neck will rebel, and so forth.

Why do these injuries occur? As we stated in the previous section, our muscles work best at a certain length. If by repetition our muscles are shortened, the ability to move through a normal arc of space is severely restricted so that normal movement patterns become impaired, sometimes imperceptibly so. Then something as simple as stepping off a curb can force that muscle to stretch too far too fast causing a strain or a tear.

Stretching enables you to counteract the constant shortening of your muscles, allowing them to retain the length from which they work best.

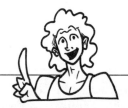

Workout Words

To **flex** means to bend, whereas to **extend** means to straighten. Flex *does not* mean contract a muscle, though you'll constantly hear it used that way in the gym.

The Basic Stretches

Stretching doesn't need to become a full-time job. Unless you're seriously considering becoming a certified yoga teacher, a few good stretches are enough to maintain your flexibility. Also, remember that you don't need to do all your stretches in the gym. Many of these can be done waiting for the train or in your office. All, however, can be done while watching TV at home.

Quadriceps

The quadriceps (quads) are the muscles on the front part of your thigh. There are four of them: rectus femoris, vastus medialis, vastus intermedius, and vastus lateralis. The rectus femoris is a two-joint muscle that *flexes* the hip and *extends* the knee. The other three are one-joint muscles that just extend the knee. Watch the Tour de France and you'll see a lot of skinny guys with overdeveloped quads.

Standing Quadriceps Stretch

1. Stand near a wall for support.

2. Bend your right leg so that that heel is moving toward your buttocks. Holding the top of your right foot with your left hand, gently pull your heel toward your butt. Make sure your knee is pointing down toward the floor.

3. Keep your shoulders and hips level.

4. Hold for 20 to 30 seconds.

5. Breathe deeply throughout the stretch and then switch to the other leg.

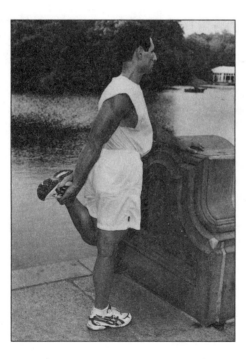

Remember to pull lightly, using your opposite hand when performing the standing quadriceps stretch.

(Source: Susanne Elstein)

Hamstrings

The hamstrings are the muscles the make up the bulk of the upper part of the back of your leg. There are three all together: biceps femoris, semitendinosis, and semi-membranosus. They are responsible for bending your knee. Olympic sprinters, NFL running backs, and thoroughbred horses have thick, highly developed "hammies." Must have something to do with running quickly, eh?

Hamstring Stretch

1. Sit and straighten your right leg.

2. Place the sole of your left foot against the inside of your right thigh.

3. Slowly bend forward from the hips toward the foot of the outstretched leg until you feel a gentle stretch.

4. Hold for 20 to 30 seconds.

5. Once the initial discomfort has diminished, bend forward a bit more.

6. Visualize your chest against your knee.

7. Hold for another 20 to 30 seconds.

As you do the hamstring stretch, avoid the temptation to push too far. Only stretch until you feel a gentle stretching sensation.

(Source: Susanne Elstein)

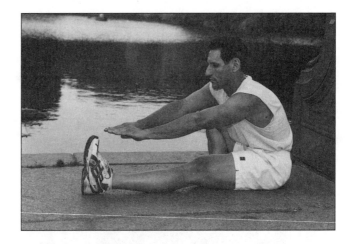

Lower and Middle Back Muscles

There are too many muscles in your lower and middle back to mention by name. Suffice it to say that if the muscles become inflexible, look out, pain will be your constant companion. Just as there are many muscles in this region, there are a number of stretches you can do.

Back and Hip Stretch

1. Lie down on an exercise mat. Bend one knee at 90° and, with your opposite hand, pull that bent leg up and over your other leg, as shown in the following figure.

2. Turn your head to look toward the hand of the arm that is straight out with palm down. (Your head should be resting on the floor, not held up.)

3. Placing the other hand on your thigh (just above the knee), pull your bent leg down toward the floor until you feel the stretch in your lower back and side of hip.

4. Keep feet and ankles relaxed and make sure the backs of your shoulders are flat on the floor.

5. Hold for 20 to 30 seconds and repeat on the other side.

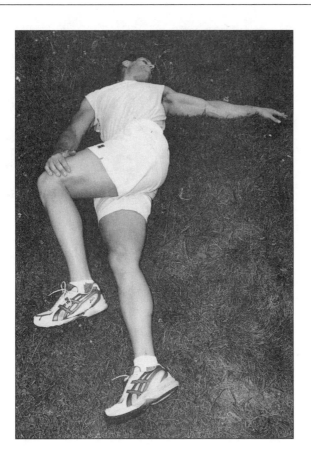

The lower back/hip stretch is a great one after a long day in an office chair.

(Source: Susanne Elstein)

Spinal Twist

1. Sit on the floor. Keep your right leg straight and cross your left leg over your right, keeping your knee pointed up toward the ceiling and your left foot just outside of your right knee.

2. Wrap your right arm around your left knee and pull your knee toward your body until you feel a stretch.

3. Twist your torso toward your left until you feel more stretch. Keep your left hand on the floor to support you as you stretch.

4. Hold the stretch for 20 to 30 seconds.

5. Repeat on the other side.

The spinal twist is another great stretch for your lower back and hips.

(Source: Susanne Elstein)

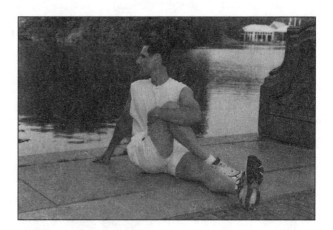

Middle Back Stretch

1. Stand and interlace your fingers out in front of you at shoulder height.

2. Turn your palms outward as you extend your arms forward as if pushing something away from you.

3. You should feel a stretch in your shoulders, middle of upper back, arms, hands, fingers, and wrists.

4. Hold for 20 to 30 seconds and repeat twice.

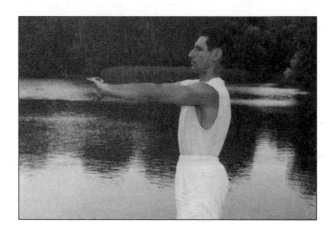

The middle back stretch helps loosen up your rhomboids and trapezius muscles.

(Source: Susanne Elstein)

Hip Flexors

The hip flexors are located on the front of the hip and, as you may have guessed, flex the hip. They are important in any activity that requires you to lift your leg—running, cycling, and stair climbing.

Lunge

1. Kneel on both knees.
2. Extend one leg forward so that the knee of the forward leg forms a right angle directly over the ankle.
3. Gently lower the front of your hip downward so that the front leg lies on the ground like an L.
4. Hold for 20 to 30 seconds.
5. Switch legs and work the other hip.

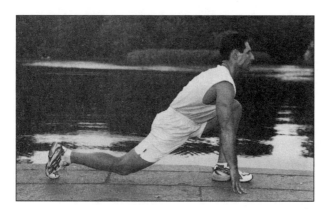

Use the lunge stretch to help increase your hip flexor flexibility.

(Source: Susanne Elstein)

Groin

Tight groin muscles are a common source of strains in sports with sudden stops, starts, and turns. The groin is defined as the depression between the thigh and the trunk and consists primarily of tendons from your adductor muscles.

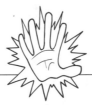

Stop Short

For any stretch where you have to bend your knee, make certain that your knee doesn't "overshoot" your toes. The knee should never be farther forward than you toes, otherwise there's too much stress on the knee.

Groin Stretch

1. Sit with your spine straight.
2. Put the soles of your feet together and grab your toes.
3. Bending from the hips, gently pull yourself forward until you feel a good stretch in your groin. Do not make the initial movement for the stretch from the head and shoulders; move from the hips. You may also feel a stretch in your lower back.
4. Hold for 20 to 30 seconds.

As your flexibility increases, you'll be able to bring your knees lower when you do the groin stretch.

(Source: Susanne Elstein)

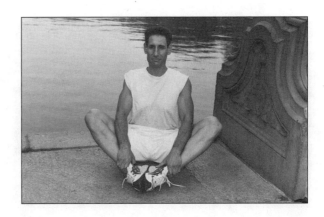

Calves

The calves are the muscles located on the lower part of the back of your leg. They help you press down on the gas pedal or rise up onto your toes to reach into the closet. There are two calf muscles: the gastrocnemius, a two-joint muscle that assists in flexing the knee as well as pointing the toes, and the soleus, a one-joint muscle that points your toes while your knee is bent.

Gastrocnemius Stretch

1. Stand on a solid support and lean forward with your hands against a wall.

2. Place one bent leg forward and extend the other leg with a straight knee behind.

3. Slowly move your hips forward, keeping your back flat. Be sure to keep the heel of the straight leg on the ground with your toes pointed straight ahead.

4. Hold for 20 to 30 seconds.

5. Don't bounce, do breathe, and repeat on the other side.

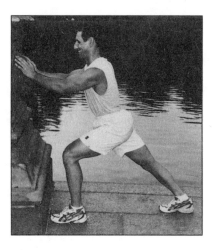

Remember to press your back heel into the ground as you do the gastrocnemius stretch.

(Source: Susanne Elstein)

Soleus Stretch

1. Begin the soleus stretch the same way you begin the gastrocnemius stretch.

2. Instead of a keeping the back leg straight, bend it until you feel a stretch in the middle part of the leg.

3. Keep your toes pointed straight ahead and your heel down.

4. Hold for 20 to 30 seconds.

5. Repeat on the other side.

The soleus stretch is similar to the gastrocnemius stretch, but your rear knee is bent.

(Source: Susanne Elstein)

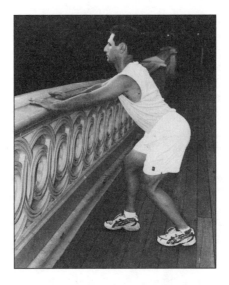

Pectorals

The pectorals (pecs) or chest muscles are extremely important to stretch because they are constantly shortened while sitting in a chair at work behind a desk, thanks to that ubiquitous slouching posture. Chippendale dancers and actors on *Baywatch* tend to have highly developed pecs.

Pec Stretch

1. Either standing or sitting on a bench, interlace your fingers behind your back.

2. With your elbows locked, lift your arms up behind you until you feel a stretch in the arms, shoulders, and chest.

3. Keep your chest out and chin in.

4. Hold for 20 to 30 seconds.

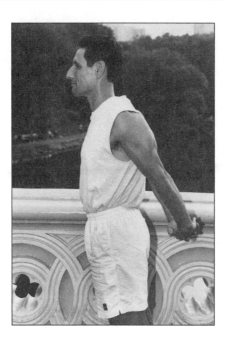

Remember to stand up straight and keep your chest high as you do the pec stretch.

(Source: Susanne Elstein)

Where Does Yoga Fit In?

When they think of yoga, many people picture a skinny bearded Indian man with no discernible spine folding himself into a human pretzel in a dimly lit room with incense burning and a sitar playing in the background. No doubt you can find that in Calcutta, but yoga has nearly become a mainstream part of our fitness culture, and it's a wonderful discipline to include in your fitness life.

Yoga classes are available at most gyms. Classes vary widely; some are more on the spiritual side and geared toward gentle stretching and relaxing. Others, like the "Power Yoga" taught by Thomas and Beryl Bender Birch in New York City, are more physically demanding and cater to the running and triathlete crowd. If you can fit a yoga class into your busy schedule—even once or twice a week—you're sure to reap big rewards.

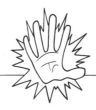

Stop Short

Is yoga for you? For many people, it can be a great, relaxing way to exercise; however, keep in mind that yoga has its limitations. While yoga may improve your strength somewhat, it's far less effective and much less efficient than pumping iron.

The Least You Need to Know

➤ No matter how tight your exercise schedule is, always find some time to stretch.

➤ Learn the stretches that are specific to your exercise routine.

➤ There is a right way and a wrong way to stretch; learn the proper technique to prevent injury.

➤ You don't have to be a yogi to benefit from yoga; it's a great way to stay limber.

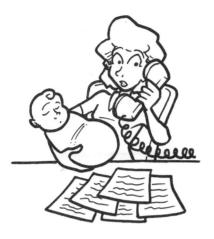

Chapter 8

Working Out with Babies and Toddlers

In This Chapter

➤ Shaping up for new moms

➤ Exercise is a family affair

➤ Rockin' and rollin' with your baby

➤ Run baby run—get fit with a jogging stroller

When experienced parents wish new parents "good luck," their intent is clearly about the little one, but they could easily be offering best wishes about the fitness challenges new parents will face given their life-altering addition.

Obviously, new mothers have more fitness issues to deal with; however, even though new fathers don't have to worry about getting back to their prepregnancy weight (at least we hope they don't), it's a solid bet that the toddler will mean a father's tight schedule just got a lot tighter.

So does parenthood mean that your fitness goals need to be put on hold until Junior goes off to college? Surely not. (If you answered "yes," you've got serious fitness issues that we need to address; if you said "no," we'll start when they go to grad school; put the book down now.) With a little fine-tuning and cagey planning, both mother and father will be able to get back on the workout bandwagon and be even fitter, more energetic parents.

Oh, Momma!

Let's take a look at the female half of the equation. Typically there are two major concerns for new mothers. First, even though kids have been around for a few years, new parents wake up and think, "Where's the instruction manual to deal with this erratically sleeping, frequently crying, constantly peeing and pooping machine?" (Admittedly, this is the less-romantic view of early childhood, but it is a dominant concern for new mothers, especially breastfeeding moms who wake up every few hours in the night.) The second less-vexing concern is "How can I get my prebaby body back?"

While we cannot tell you why babies don't come with instruction manuals, we can give you plenty of tips on getting back into shape and figuring out how to work out even if you're a new parent. Luckily, nature has provided us *Homo sapiens* with a few

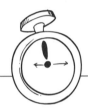

Short Cuts

One of the best ways to begin a postpartum fitness program is to hook up with other new mothers who are eager to get back into working out. Not only is it a great way to forge friendships with other women facing similar challenges, but scheduling a workout together ensures that you're far less likely to skip your workout.

neat tricks. Typically, a woman gains between 30 and 40 pounds by the time she delivers a baby. Of course, many of those pounds are shed when the baby leaves mom's womb for a hospital room. Afterward, it's best to nurse your baby, since breastfeeding mothers burn through calories the way Elizabeth Taylor goes through husbands. (Breastfeeding requires more calories than being pregnant.)

So in fact, for new, breastfeeding mothers the key isn't so much losing weight as it is regaining muscle tone. Of course, if you've been exercising throughout your pregnancy—and you should—you'll be better able to jump back on the workout wagon. Either way, an oft-overlooked point when it comes to regaining your former figure is to exercise extreme patience. With all huge life changes, you need to regain your strength, establish a routine with the new kid, and only then start thinking about working out. In the interim, eat a healthful diet, walk with Junior, and remain patient. Before you can say lactation consultant, we'll have you back in the gym pumping iron again instead of breast milk.

To state the obvious, pregnancy plays havoc with your body. Not only have you gained two dozen or more pounds, your muscles have been stretched like a bloated hot water bottle and your energy reserve severely sapped. In other words, please don't expect to bounce right back and start scaling mountains. The first few months of tending to a baby is mountain enough. It will take some time for your hormones to get back under control and your muscles to regain strength. Start slowly and with consistency you can restart your prepregnancy exercise routine with the little one in tow.

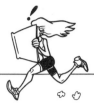

Info to Go

Since it took your body nine months to produce a child, it's unrealistic to expect to lose the extra weight in a few weeks. On the other hand, there's no reason that you can't be back to your fighting weight within two to three months. While some experts advise losing two pounds or more per week until you return to your desired weight, we think this is too much pressure to put on yourself. The key is to follow general weight-loss principles—burn more calories than you consume—and you're on your way. Once you resume exercising, your body (and time) will take care of the extra weight.

The Big Comeback

There are a host of factors that determine how soon you can resume exercising after your baby is born. If you exercised throughout your pregnancy, have an uncomplicated vaginal delivery, and you feel up to it, then you can probably return to exercise two to four weeks after the big day. The key here is to be true to your instinct. If you're not up for returning to the gym, you can begin doing isometric abdominal and pelvic floor exercises immediately after delivery to speed up the healing process. You can also begin a regular walking routine at a moderate pace as soon as your caregiver gives you the okay.

Since your baby requires a lot of attention and takes precedence over all else, you may have to be creative about how and where you sneak in your workouts. If you have child care, this is fairly easy; if you don't, you need to be more motivated. However, nothing puts a baby to sleep faster than motion. If you stuff the little one into a snugly or backpack and hit the road, you're likely to inspire a nap and get a workout in at the same time. The fresh air will do you and your upstart a world of good.

We have a female friend who used to set up her stationary bike next to her infant's crib and cycle for a few minutes each time he took a nap. Not only did she get to work out, the snoozing tot

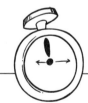

Short Cuts

Ironically, sometimes the time we feel like exercising the least is when we need to do it most. As a result, try to be active every day, even if you only walk around the block once or twice.

seemingly slept securely knowing his mom was close by. We used to joke that if she had been able to hook up a gizmo to connect the cycling with rocking the cradle, the baby might never had woken up and she'd have become a world-class cyclist.

Start Me Up

In addition to improving overall conditioning, there are some basic isometric exercises that can help target muscles that are directly affected during the pregnancy and delivery.

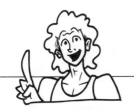

Workout Words

Kegel exercises, named after Dr. Arnold Kegel, are a technique to strengthen the muscles of the pelvic wall.

Strengthening the Pelvic Wall

The *Kegel exercises* aren't going to make their way into aerobic classes any time soon, but they will help to strengthen your vaginal and pelvic walls. The way to visualize doing it correctly is to think of starting and stopping the flow of urine as you go to the bathroom.

1. Lie on your back with your knees bent.

2. Begin squeezing, holding each contraction for a two-second count.

3. Do one set of 10, working your way up to three sets of 10 to 12 over the next week.

Audacious Abdominals

The most common complaint we hear from new mothers is, "I just had a baby so why do I look as though I'm still pregnant?" Don't fret; follow the abdominal routine below and you'll have your tummy back to its former self.

1. Lie on your back with your knees bent.

2. Inhale deeply through your nose. As you exhale through your mouth, think about pressing your belly button down toward the floor, tightening your abdominal muscles as you do so.

3. Hold for a three-count and inhale as you release your muscles. Do one set of 10, working your way up to three sets of 10 to 15 over the next two weeks.

If you've had a vaginal delivery, your doctor will probably tell you that you can begin to do crunches after two weeks. If you had a C-section, it's usually more like four weeks.

Tighten Those Gluteals

If your buttock muscles have become a little flabby, we've got an exercise to strengthen your rear end.

1. Lie on your back with your legs straight.

2. Inhale deeply through your nose. As you exhale through your mouth, squeeze your buttocks together tightly. Hold the contraction for a five-count and release as you inhale.

3. Do one set of 10, working your way up to three sets of 10 to 15 over the next two weeks.

After the second week, you can begin doing modified squats and lunges.

Joining a Postpartum Class

Another good way to get into shape is to join mom and baby classes, which are especially designed for new mothers. Not only will they help you get fitter, you'll be able to tap into the community of like-minded new mothers. Also, don't underestimate the importance of making an appointment to get out of the house. Often new mother's find most of a day has passed and they've not made it out the door. This is fine if it pleases you, but string a few of these days together and you're likely to be climbing the walls.

As your child gets older, you can incorporate game playing into your fitness goals: playing tag, sprinting, jumping rope, splashing in a shallow kiddie pool.

Stop Short

Make sure that a certified aerobics instructor trained in postpartum fitness teaches the class. The class should emphasize low-impact aerobics with simple choreography, strength training, and flexibility exercises to reduce the risk of muscular injury.

Baby, Let's Stroll

Strollercize is a system of exercise developed by personal trainer Elizabeth Trindade in 1990. After the birth of her first child, her husband gave her a "big, clunky" stroller. With creative energy and ingenuity, she developed a program consisting of cardiovascular, strengthening, and flexibility exercises that are done with baby and stroller. In 1992 the system she created received medical approval and in 1993 Strollercize classes began in New York City's Central Park. It is now licensed in New Jersey, Washington, D.C., North Carolina, Massachusetts, and Illinois.

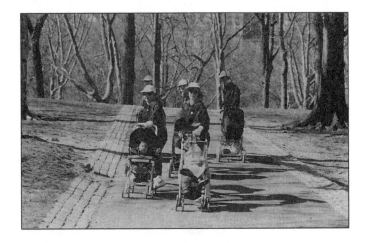

A group of new moms taking a Strollercize class in New York's Central Park.

Two for One

Here's a news flash: Becoming a new parent is a wonderful experience wrought with joy, happiness, confusion, frustration, and fatigue. Without a doubt, parenthood is a two- (or more) person job. Given this, mutual support and understanding are essential. A great way to accomplish this is to participate in an exercise routine together.

"Good idea," you're thinking, "now who takes care of the new little one?" If it is logistically impossible to go to a health club together, don't despair; we'll give you some tips on putting together an exercise routine you can do at home.

Cardio Partner Time

If you have enough room in your home, you can buy cardiovascular exercise equipment that you both can use at the same time. No, we don't recommend both of you running on a treadmill together—that's taking togetherness a bit too far. But you can follow the lead of our friends who own a treadmill, Stairclimber, and stationary bike. Frequently, when their three-year-old boy hits the hay, they'll hop on one of the above-mentioned pieces of equipment and exercise together for 20 to 30 minutes. If your child is considerably younger, you can take turns. It is best to devise a system that works out the logistics of who attends the snoozer should he or she wake up before the allotted workout time is over.

Strength Training with Your Partner

A great way to exercise together is to strength train by literally opposing each other. While it sounds goofy, using the resistance of your partner, you can replicate virtually any exercise that you can do in a gym. Manual resistance exercises are also a great way for a couple to encourage each other to exercise and participate in each other's fitness. Jonathan used these techniques extensively when he worked as a personal trainer and is still a strong advocate of the technique. Manual resistance allows you to work any muscle you can think of, at any angle you like, and you don't have to worry about moving from machine to machine or changing weights.

Working Out with Baby

If you are fortunate enough to be able to go to the gym, pick one with a baby-sitting facility. Most health clubs require that the child be at least two years old unless there are classes specifically for new moms and their babies. Dads can go and give Mom a chance to rest at home. Moms can go if Dad is at home and there is no baby-sitter. This way, new parents can get a bit of sorely needed quiet time alone.

If you do find a gym that offers child care for infants, it's important that you go check out the sitter and the space before you work out there. Observe how he or she interacts with the other children. Remember, trust your instincts on how you feel about this person. If you like her, it's a good idea to get your child familiar with the person and space before leaving them alone— otherwise you may spend most of your workout time running from the gym to your crying child. While this might be a good workout, it's not terribly relaxing.

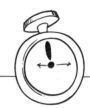

Short Cuts

Initially, men think that they won't get a good workout simply because their partner is a woman. But the truth is that this routine works equally well whether your workout partner is a man or woman. In Chapter 10, "The 15-Minute Strength-Training Workout," we'll show you a host of manual resistance exercises for every muscle group you own—as well as a few you didn't know you had.

Rocking Out with Your Baby

We once read somewhere that a great way for a new mom and baby to bond was to spend some quality time working out together. As hardened cynics, we pictured the drooling infant holding a stopwatch in his or her chubby hand, shouting, "Fast, Mom, pick it up into a higher fat-burning zone." What the author meant, of course, was that spending time with her infant doing something the mother enjoys is a good way to improve Mom's mental and physical health—an incalculable benefit to all involved.

As we mentioned, the best option is a nice, brisk walk—an age-old exercise that is usually invigorating, stamina-building, and fat-burning all at the same time.

A Bicycle Built for Mom and Baby

We know a woman who was the number-one ranked road cyclist in Montana who had her eye on the 1988 U.S. Olympic Trials. A year before the race, she became pregnant and had a baby girl. Instead of compromising her dream, as soon as she was up to it, she set her new little training partner in a bike trailer and trained like a madwoman. Ironically (or not), she became fitter fast. So much so, in fact, that many of her unencumbered teammates starting pulling weighted wagons as well.

Baby seats come in two types—front or rear mount—while trailers put the child at ground level behind your bike. We recently read about a family of five—mother, dad, and three kids—who cycled across the United States on a rather ingenious bicycle built for four—with the youngest riding comfortably in a trailer. Ambitious, no doubt, but doable.

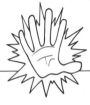

Stop Short

All new mothers suffer from sleep deprivation; yet many of the fitness-oriented moms we know try to get in their exercise while the little one is snoozing. Good intention, but that's just when you should be napping as well. Instead of burning the candle at both ends, try putting your wakeful baby in a baby sling and go for a long walk. As your endurance and stamina build, increase the distance or add hillier terrain. If you're lucky, the walk will put the child to sleep and you can then get some shut-eye yourself when you get home.

Baby Bicycle Seats

As we just mentioned, baby seats are attached to either the back of the bicycle (the most common) or the front. Most are recommended for children eight months of age or up to 40 pounds. Check with the individual manufacturers for the specifics. Most are outfitted with a padded seat, armrests, and adjustable footrests along with a lap and shoulder harness. No matter which model you buy, start slowly and get your infant used to the idea—even have him or her sit in it a few times inside without pedaling at all. Start slowly and you'll be able to go further, longer, later.

According to the journal *The Physician and Sports Medicine,* while rear-mounted baby seats are more popular, the safety of the front-mounted seats is preferred. The journal points to the improved stability and balance of the front mounts as well as the ability for the parent and child to communicate more easily. If you use a rear-mounted one, make sure that the child's hands are well shielded from the wheel and exercise caution when climbing out of the saddle, as there will be an unusual shift of weight to the rear of the bike.

Most manufacturers recommend their seats for children as young as 9 to 12 months, though you should check with your (child's) pediatrician. The main concern is your child's ability to maintain proper head and neck control. The capacity of most seats is 30 to 40 pounds. After that, a trailer is the way to go.

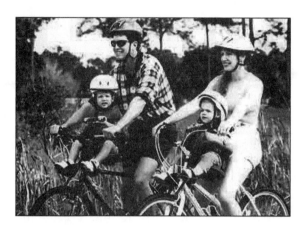

Two bikes with baby seats and four helmets add up safe family fun.

Baby Trailers

Baby trailers are basically strollers that you can hook up to your bicycle. Keep the following in mind before you head out the door with your precious cargo.

➤ Always use shoulder and lap belts on the child.

➤ Avoid busy streets whenever possible.

➤ Give yourself room to stop. Braking distance increases and braking control decreases with loads.

➤ With the additional width of the trailer, be careful taking turns.

➤ Practice using the trailer without the child to get used to the feel of the attachment. When you take your child out for the first time, make sure it is in an area that is not busy.

➤ Baby trailers are not for newborns; tots must be at least one year old before you can exercise safely with them.

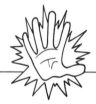

Stop Short

Always put a helmet on your child whenever you hit the road with the baby trailer or on the bicycle seats. Go to a bike shop to make sure that the fit is appropriate. There are lots of fun-looking helmets that your kids are bound to enjoy. And while you are there, make sure you get one for yourself.

It's ironic that many parents would never put their child in a bike seat or trailer without a hard-shell helmet, but they won't wear one themselves. The reasoning being, apparently, that they won't crash. Such logic actually suggests a past blow to the head. It summons the old cyclist adage: The only people who don't wear helmets are the ones with nothing worth protecting.

Jog, Baby

As any New Yorker can tell you, baby joggers are extremely popular. Initially, when Deidre began training for the 1999 New York City Marathon, she thought it delightful that Prospect Park was full of jogging parents pushing their children around the park. As she got fitter, however, she developed a healthy disdain for the parent/child teams that were moving faster than she was. One woman in particular named Barbara Brewer even passed speedy men while pushing her little one. Of course, Barbara, one of the toughest women we've laid eyes on, clocked subseven-minute miles with her newborn as she trained for the World Duathlon Championships. (A duathlon is a triathlon without the swim—run/bike/run.)

Baby joggers are basically idiot proof, but there are a few things to keep in mind. While some manufacturers say it's safe for infants as young as six to eight weeks, some pediatricians recommend six months. Weight limitations depend on the jogger itself. Be careful not to exceed the suggested weight limit, because it can cause the stroller to tip. And remember, as tempting as it may be, don't try and cajole your child into pushing you.

Questions you need to ask about the stroller you choose:

1. Does it fold?
2. Can it be adjusted for height?
3. Is it safe?
4. Is there a lifetime warranty?

Here are a few other factors to consider when purchasing a baby jogger. Do you enjoy running on pavement or off road? Generally speaking, the larger the wheels are, the more suitable for off-road jogging they are (although we don't recommend taking your child off road, as it may be too bumpy for your precious cargo). Wheels range from 12 inches to 20 inches in diameter, with 12 inches the most suitable for pavement and 20 inches suitable for the serious off-road runner. Sixteen-inch wheels are suitable for rougher surfaces such as snow and sand. In addition, wheels can be smooth or textured, with smooth wheels for pavement and textured wheels for off road.

The Least You Need to Know

➤ Being new parents can be a wonderful, trying time, but there are ways to keep your fitness intact.

➤ You can create a stronger bond with your little one by working out together.

➤ Health clubs with baby-sitting can give new parents much needed quiet time.

➤ Postpartum exercise classes are a great way for new moms to get to know one another.

Part 3

The Workouts: 15 Minutes to 30 Minutes

Enough talk about time management and the benefits of exercise—now it's time to get to work. Fifteen or thirty minutes may not seem like a lot of time, but this part will present you with a variety of ideas of how to make the most of your exercise: in the gym, on the road, or at home.

We'll discuss how to break a sweat in just 15 minutes and give you strategies for getting strong in that same time frame. We'll progress up to 30 minutes of cardio and then outline strengthening routines you can do in half an hour.

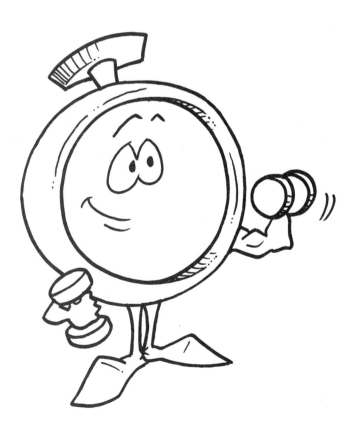

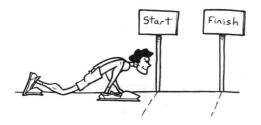

Chapter 9

The 15-Minute Cardio Workout

In This Chapter

➤ Walk this way—power walking instead of jogging

➤ Jumping rope for fitness

➤ Stairclimbing is a challenging workout

➤ Circuit training helps build muscle and stamina

Pick up one of the many fitness magazines on the newsstands and you're bound to see exaggerated claims of "Lose 10 pounds in a week in only 15 minutes a day!" (Not eating for a week might help you lose 10 pounds, but we don't recommend it.) Please heed this warning: Run, don't walk, from any article or infomercial that makes such bold claims. Still, that doesn't mean that with a little creativity, you can't break a sweat and be productive.

As someone's sage grandmother once said, "It's the drops in the bucket that make a big puddle." Even if you only have 15 minutes to squeeze in a workout, you'll be improving your fitness compared to doing nothing at all. No, it's not enough time to transform you into a fitness model, but there are several techniques you can do to help you release stress, burn calories, and build muscle. In this chapter we'll provide you with several ideas of quick things you can do away from the gym.

Left Foot, Right Foot

Let's get simple. The easiest, most basic thing you can do in 15 minutes to improve your fitness is to go for a *power walk*. No, power walking doesn't mean you talk on your cell phone while making business calls. And power walking isn't running. Nor is it a leisurely stroll where you window shop along the way—that's just not going to cut it in terms of caloric expenditure or health gains. And the final "not," power walking

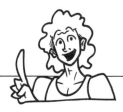

Workout Words

So what *is* it? **Power walking** is brisk, purposeful walking. You go as fast as you can, but you keep one foot on the ground at all times, (as opposed to jogging, where you get airborne), and swing your arms forcefully.

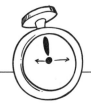

Short Cuts

Think 60 seconds of jumping rope is easy? The world record for most jumps in one minute is 292. That's almost five revolutions per second!

also isn't race walking, the Olympic sport that would garner you some very strange stares along the way.

Think of the pace you'd walk if you were going to the movies and didn't want to miss the opening credits (a moderate pace, right?). Now consider your speed if you were about to miss your flight to The Bahamas (double time, we're guessing).

While this walking stuff seems too easy or basic to be useful, consider the fact that "walking clubs" and classes are popping up all over the country. In fact, Jake Jacobson, author of *Healthwalk to Fitness* and considered "the father of health walking," says that if you walk at a good clip for 15 minutes you can burn about 100 calories. (A good benchmark will be to see if you can cover one mile in that time.) Plus, power walking doesn't require any equipment. (Speaking of which, don't bother with hand weights as you walk—they can throw off your stride and possibly increase your blood pressure.) And while 100 calories might not seem like a lot, the stress reduction is impossible to calculate. Walking with purpose (or just walking in general) clears your head and improves your circulation and digestion. Get really good at it and you might not have to break into a trot when you're late for your next flight.

Jump Rope: Not Just for Kids and Boxers

One of the most valuable, yet inexpensive and portable pieces of equipment is the jump rope. Jumping rope has been a useful training tool for everyone from boxers to martial artists to runners to basketball players. (If you want to see some real athleticism, come to Brooklyn and watch a group of girls shred the sidewalk using two ropes at once.) Not only are ropes cheap, they fit neatly into a briefcase or backpack and you need a modest amount of floor space and a high ceiling to skip away.

Here are the top-four reasons to jump rope:

1. It will improve your cardiovascular endurance.
2. Estimates are that you'll burn as much as 200 calories in just 15 minutes. (And the bigger you are, the more calories you'll burn while jumping.)

3. You'll help tone your thighs, calves, and even your upper body.

4. Rope jumping can help your coordination, balance, and agility.

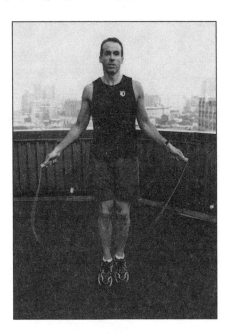

Jonathan at work jumping rope.

Let's take a look at the basics of jumping rope.

Choosing a Rope

The proper rope length depends on how tall you are. According to jumprope.com, here's how you figure out how long of a rope to use.

Length	Suitable for Height
7'	up to 4'10"
8'	4'10"–5'3"
9'	5'4"–5'10"
10'	5'11" or over

Types of Rope

Beaded ropes are relatively inexpensive and durable. On the downside, they aren't very fast, so if you're a skilled jumper you may want something else. Woven ropes are lightweight and as a result it's hard to get them moving quickly. While they're great for the abrasive pavement of a schoolyard, they're not our favorites.

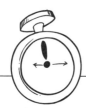

Short Cuts

Jump ropes are available at most sporting goods stores. Try them before you buy to ensure that you choose the right length and weight.

Rubber ropes have distinct pros and cons—all of which Jonathan learned the hard way. The good news is that because they're heavy, they're fast. The bad news is that when you get them rolling and you miss, it really hurts. Jonathan refers to his rubber rope as the "negative reinforcement rope." Despite the repeated blows to his shins, Jonathan never goes on a road trip without his trusty rope, since you never know what the weather will be or if your flight will be delayed. As long as a fitness fiend has a rope, he's well armed.

Our favorite rope is the leather or vinyl speed rope. It's heavy enough to get some good speed, but not so much that your upper body gets too tired from spinning the rope. If you get one with a good pair of handles with ball bearings, you'll be flying.

Whichever type of rope you choose, here's a jump rope workout:

➤ Do a quick warm-up of some light "ropeless" jumping.

➤ The basic jump is with both legs, pushing off and landing on the balls of your feet. Keep your arms at your side, just above your waist.

➤ As you progress, you can try advanced techniques such as double jumps, in which the rope rotates twice while you're airborne. This obviously requires you to use more leg power, but also puts your upper body to work more than single jumps. Start off by adding an occasional double mixed in with your singles.

➤ Crossovers will impress your friends and spice up the workout. There's no need to break your jumping cadence—just bring your arms inward and cross the rope in front of you.

➤ Single-leg hops are a good way to vary your workout. Try alternating legs, or do several repeated hops per leg to give your calves an extra workout.

Jump Rope Tips

Jump only high enough to clear the rope. Many people leap too high and exhaust themselves after just a minute or two.

Keep your wrists close to your body as you spin the rope.

Wear good sneakers—quality cross-trainers are best. Running shoes elevate your heel a little too much, though they'll do if necessary.

Land gently on the balls of your feet without locking your knees.

Stand tall. If you have to duck to get under the rope, it's either too short or you're holding your arms too low.

If you become good at jumping, you may even want to attend one of the many jumping classes that are popping up at Crunch, Bally's, and other gyms around the country.

Upstairs, Downstairs

If rope jumping doesn't seem challenging enough for you, we've got another good quick workout idea. Every year Jonathan competes in the annual 86-story Empire State Building run, and if you were to ask him, say, after the eleventh floor how he felt, he'd tell you that 15 minutes of stair climbing is more than enough time to push even the best athlete. (Actually, he wouldn't tell you since he's huffing and puffing too hard to say boo.) Don't worry, we're not suggesting that you jump right in and try to tackle the Empire State Building—any five-story building will do just fine.

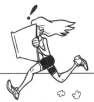

Info to Go

A few years ago, Jonathan participated in a 40-story stair climb race to raise money for the Cystic Fibrosis Foundation. The following year he recruited members from his gym. One ambitious woman in her 50s who signed up had started exercising only months earlier, after her doctor told her to work out or pay the piper. Initially she was only able to climb a few flights of stairs with breaks after each flight. She soon progressed to two or three continuous flights. In no time she was taking the stairs to her fifth-floor office rather than the elevator. Four months later on race day, she found herself high atop New York's 40-story World Financial Center under her own power.

It's funny how many people will go flog themselves silly at a gym lifting weights or on the Stairmaster, but they dread the idea of climbing even a couple of flights of real stairs. How often have you seen someone sprint down a long hallway to catch an elevator to avoid climbing one or two flights of stairs?

Of course we want you to use the stairs in lieu of the elevator whenever possible—remember to take your fitness outside of the gym and you'll get fitter faster. However, if you have 10 or 15 minutes and want to get a real workout, don a pair of running shoes and get ready to climb.

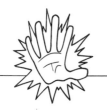

Stop Short

Stair climbing is a killer workout, so make sure you warm up well and stretch out your calves with both the gastrocnemius and soleus stretches we showed you back in Chapter 7, "Start with Stretching"; that is, unless you appreciate excruciating muscle soreness the day after your workout.

Just in case you were wondering, stair-climb racers generally take the steps two at a time and pull hard on the banisters. Unless you're racing or have an angry mob chasing you, one step at a time will do fine when you're getting started. Lightly hold the handrail and try to climb at a steady pace. Strike the step with the middle of your foot and roll forward onto your toes as you pull yourself up. As your conditioning improves, you'll be able to take two steps at a time.

Obviously the size of the building you're in will dictate the length of your climb. If you only have 5 or 10 flights, you can climb them, scoot back downstairs, and take another "lap." If it's practical, try taking the elevator back downstairs. Sound strange? Descending the stairs puts a lot more stress on your quads and knees and can lead to excessive soreness without any real benefit. If you have to use the stairs to get down, walk; don't run. In addition, most times you can get back to the ground floor (and back to climbing) quicker if you take the elevator.

Short Circuit

Circuit training, a lifting regimen that gained popularity a couple of decades ago, is still going strong in some circles. You're probably wondering why we're mentioning lifting weights in a chapter on cardiovascular training. Because the benefits of circuit training are both increased cardiovascular training and strength. By quickly moving from one weight station to another—ideally limiting the time between exercises to 30 seconds—you not only strengthen your muscles, but you also enjoy a cardiovascular training effect.

Sounds great, right? The problem is that as exercise goes, circuit training falls under the category of jack-of-all-trades, but master of none. Here's why. The short rest between sets are great for saving time, but prevents you from fully recovering and recruiting as much muscle as possible when lifting. Also, while your heart rate does remain elevated throughout such a workout, the physiological mechanism that causes your heart to pump rapidly during weight lifting is different than the mechanism that raises your heart rate when you go for a run or step on the StairMaster. That's because when you go for a run or a ride, not only does your heart rate increase, but so does your stroke volume, the amount of blood ejected from your heart with each beat. When you lift, your heart rate goes up, but your stroke volume stays stable, and sometimes even decreases. In other words, 140 beats is not always the same as 140 beats. If this were true, watching scary movies or riding roller coasters would also qualify as cardio work.

That said, if you have just 15 minutes to spare, circuit training is a good quick workout since it improves both your muscular and cardiovascular systems. Since we're assuming that your 15-minute workout is taking place away from the gym, the routine we're outlining uses dumbbells or resistance bands (which we'll discuss further in the next chapter). We especially like the Power Block dumbbells that we mentioned in Chapter 6, "Strengthening," for circuit training. The ability to quickly change the weight allows you to keep the rest between sets to a minimum, thus getting the maximum benefit from your circuit training. Whether you use dumbbells or bands, either one can be easily stored in your home or office. Both routines require no other equipment or benches.

Choose a weight (or in the case of resistance bands, choose the appropriate resistance) for each exercise that allows you to complete between 12 and 15 reps without sacrificing form. Remember that maintaining good form is key—don't let the fast pace of the circuit translate to sloppy technique and fast movements.

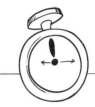

Short Cuts

While circuit training does improve your strength, it doesn't do so nearly as much as more conventional strength-training methods. In addition, the cadiovascular benefits are not nearly as significant as those gained from running, cycling, or other standard methods.

Ten exercises at about a minute each with 30 seconds recovery allows time for 10 exercises in 15 minutes.

Dumbbell or resistance band circuit

Lateral raise	Military press
Lunges (dumbbells) or leg press (bands)	Biceps curl
Standing calf raises	Triceps extension
Chest press (lie on the floor)	Crunch
Bent row (one arm at a time)	Upright row

Remember that your workouts don't have to be an all-or-nothing proposition. Sure, you'd be better off going for a long run or bike ride than squeezing in 15 minutes. However, as we've told you before, 15 minutes is far better than nothing—for both your body and your mind. As the world-class multisport athlete Steve Ilg says, "Fitness training improves not only your physical well-being but also your determination. You are developing inner strength in addition to outer strength." In other words, even if you don't have 30 minutes or more to spare, don't blow off a good opportunity to squeeze in a short but effective 15-minute workout. With a little creativity and ambition, you can gain significant mental and physical benefits from even the briefest of workouts.

The Least You Need to Know

➤ Purposeful walking can be an effective activity if you have limited time.

➤ Jumping rope isn't only for young girls. Elite athletes do it for superior cardio-vascular training.

➤ Climbing stairs is not as easy as you think. Make a habit of it and see your fitness gains increase dramatically.

➤ While some think of circuit training in cardiovascular terms, we think of it in purely timesaving terms.

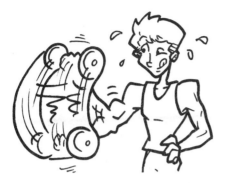

Chapter 10

The 15-Minute Strength-Training Workout

In This Chapter

➤ Give us 15 minutes and we'll give you a basic and sound foundation

➤ Resistance bands when the choices are slim

➤ Manual resistance routines for two

➤ Calisthenics are not only for the military

Let's get the bad news out of the way first. If you aspire to become Mr. or Ms. Olympia (or even runner-up), 15 minutes of strength training is not enough. Now the good news: A well-conceived quarter hour worth of lifting could help you maintain or even gain strength. (Just for the record: 15 minutes is plenty of time to do a thorough abdominal and lower back routine.) In this chapter, we'll show you several different strategies for using that limited time—using everything from calisthenics to rubber bands to resistance provided by a workout partner.

In addition, for those of you who don't have time to get to the gym but can dedicate a few minutes each day to lifting, we'll lay out a routine that you can do with just a set of dumbbells and a weight bench in the comfort and privacy of your own home.

Band on the Run

In the physical therapist's office they're called TheraBands; in the "toning" class at the gym they're DynaBands; or you can just go by the generic name of resistance bands. Whatever you call them, resistance bands are basically a lot like rubber bands on steroids. And while the name may sound like a subversive group of terrorists, the variety we're talking about are giant rubber bands that comprise a color-coded progressive resistance system. Included are accessories such as exercise handles and door anchors to make the exercises more versatile. These accessories enable you to work out with the bands with greater stability.

Pros of resistance bands:

➤ Easy to pack

➤ Variable resistance

➤ Can be used for a variety of exercises

➤ Safe

Cons of resistance bands:

➤ The resistance is not constant throughout the full range of motion (ROM).

➤ While there are some good exercises to do for the smaller body parts like shoulders and arms, there are not many effective exercises to do for larger body parts like your glutes, quads, and hamstrings.

➤ There is a limit to their shelf life; the more you use them, the more worn they get, leading to breaks in the band.

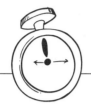

Short Cuts

The best thing about these resistance bands is their portability and relative efficiency when you're on the road (or even in your office if you have time to spare). While we're not saying that you can get in great shape using them on a daily basis, their convenience is their biggest selling point. While they won't take the place of 100-pound dumbbells, they can help give your muscles a workout.

Deidre doing biceps curls with resistance bands.

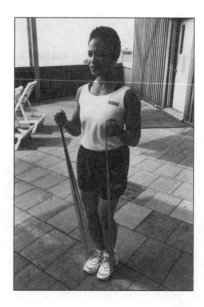

The trick to using resistance bands is to use a band with the right amount of resistance, and to have some tension on the band as you start the exercise. Having the proper tension helps you to gain strength at the beginning of the range of motion. If you want to get fancy use more than one resistance band at a time. Doubling up can make an exercise particularly challenging even if you're already strong.

Here are several exercises you can do with resistance bands:

Legs

Seated leg press: Sit on a step or bench with your knee bent. Wrap the resistance band around one foot, and grasp both ends in each hand. Keep your toes pointed slightly downward. Slowly straighten your leg (don't lock your knee). Slowly return to the starting position.

Back

Seated rows: Sit on the floor and wrap the resistance band around the balls of both feet. With elbows bent, pull your arms back while squeezing your shoulder blades together. Slowly return to the starting position.

Chest

Chest press: Wrap the resistance band around your back. Grip the band ends with both hands and press your arms forward. Slowly return to the starting position.

Shoulders

Lateral raises: Stand with feet shoulder width apart and place one end of the resistance band under your foot as you hold the other end in your hand. Slowly raise your arm out to the side until you reach shoulder height. Slowly return to the starting position.

Front raises: Same starting position. Slowly raise your arm upward until you reach shoulder height. Slowly return to the starting position.

Biceps

Biceps curls: Stand with your feet shoulder width apart and place one end of the resistance band under your foot as you hold the other end in your hand. Slowly curl your arm by bending your elbow toward your shoulder. Slowly return to the starting position.

Triceps

Triceps extensions: Place a towel around your neck. Place the resistance band along the towel. Grip both ends in each hand so that your elbows are close to your body as you slowly straighten your arms. Make sure to keep your wrists straight. Slowly return to the starting position.

Here's an efficient 15-minute workout that you can do with resistance bands. Try to find a band that will allow you to do between 12 and 15 good repetitions. For the abdominal exercises (where you can't easily adjust the resistance as you would with a band or a weight), that number may vary. Still, don't worry about trying to do a million reps. If you focus on good form, you'll be pressing to do more than 15 or so reps.

Body Part	Exercise
Legs/hips	Leg press
Back	Seated row
Chest	Chest press
Shoulders	Lateral raise
Arms	Biceps curl
	Triceps extension
Midsection	Reverse crunches
	Crunches

Since this is the first time we've introduced crunches and reverse crunches into the mix, let's go over proper form for these exercises. While they're gym staples, it doesn't mean that they're always performed properly.

Here's the proper start/ finish position for the crunch.

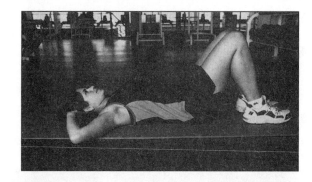

Note that the lower back remains pressed into the floor and her shoulder blades are off the mat.

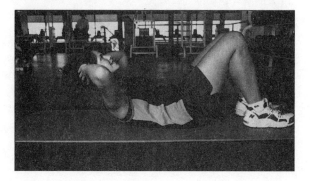

Crunch Time

Crunches are the definitive abdominal exercise—sort of the sit-up of the twenty-first century. This exercise helps you develop the muscles that create the much-sought-after "six-pack." You can vary your hand position to make the exercise harder or easier. The easiest variation is to put your hands straight at your sides with your fingers pointing toward your toes. Crossing your arms over your chest makes it a little more challenging. Lightly lacing your fingers behind your neck makes the exercise harder still. If you really want to make it tough, holding a light weight behind your head will make the exercise extra challenging.

Regardless of your hand position, here's the drill:

1. Lie on a mat with your knees bent and your feet flat on the floor.

2. Tighten your abdominal muscles and slowly curl your torso up for a three-second count until your shoulder blades are off the mat.

3. Pause for a second and slowly lower yourself to your starting position for three seconds.

Crunch Tips

Imagine a tennis ball between your chin and your chest. Maintain that space rather than tucking your chin as you curl up. Focusing your eyes on a point on the ceiling makes it easier to do this.

If you choose the hands-behind-the-head method, keep your elbows back, rather than flapping them forward.

Come up to about a 30° angle. There's no reason to come higher.

Keep your lower back pressed into the mat at all times. This will help protect your back and make the exercise more effective.

Exhale forcefully on the way up and inhale as you return to the starting position.

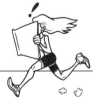

Info to Go

Crunches and other abdominal exercises are a great way to strengthen your muscles, but even doing hundreds of reps won't burn fat in your midsection (or anywhere else for that matter).

Reverse Crunches

Reverse crunches, which work the lower section of your abdominals (the bottom two of the six-pack), are not nearly as impressive looking as other so-called lower abdominal exercises such as leg raises and "bicycles," but they are safer and more effective.

Here's the skinny on the reverse crunch:

1. Lie on a mat with your legs up in the air with a slight bend in your knees. Think of yourself as a giant letter *L*.

2. Rest your arms at your sides.

3. Keep your head on the mat and tighten your abdominal muscles.

4. Lift your butt off the floor so that your legs go up and slightly back toward your head for a count of three. Exhale forcefully as you rise.

5. Pause at the top and slowly return to the starting position while inhaling.

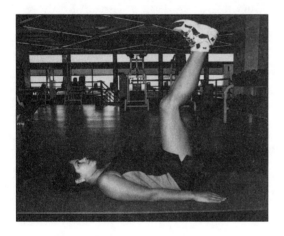

The proper start/finish position for the reverse crunch.

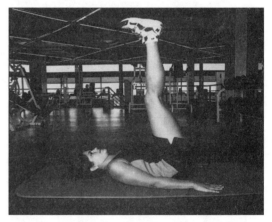

In the reverse crunch middle position, the lower back remains pressed into the mat as the heels press up.

A Helping Hand

Good old manual resistance is a solid tactic to work your muscles when there's no equipment around. To do these exercises, however, requires another human being. Manual resistance exercises, or manuals, involve your workout partner creating the resistance by applying force against you. While equipment isn't needed to get a good manual workout, you might want to add high-tech, state-of-the-art tools such as a towel or a broomstick to help you make some of these exercises more effective.

In 1997 Jonathan, a near-professional skeptic, took a workshop with John Philbin, an assistant strength coach for the NFL's Washington Redskins and president of the National Sports Performance Association (NSPA). Philbin demonstrated how strength coaches and personal trainers can employ manual resistance with a wide variety of clients. After demonstrating exercises for every body part on a variety of people, Philbin had convinced Jonathan.

According to the NSPA, here are the advantages of manual resistance exercises:

➤ No equipment is needed.

➤ You can do it anywhere.

➤ It's an effective substitute for normal routines.

➤ The speed of exercise can be controlled.

Their list of disadvantages includes:

➤ You need two people.

➤ It requires skill to be a good spotter.

➤ The spotter must be aware of the lifter's capability.

➤ You can't measure strength gains.

➤ The lifter may be significantly stronger than the spotter.

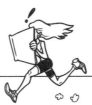

Info to Go

The positive or concentric phase of an exercise is the lifting phase. The muscle's force is greater than the resistance, so the muscle shortens to move the weight. In the eccentric or negative phase, the weight is returned to its starting position as the resistance overcomes the force that the muscle exerts.

Here are a few manual resistance exercises you can do in 15 minutes:

Body Part	Exercise
Legs/hips	Leg extension
	Leg curl

continues

continued

Body Part	Exercise
Back	Lat pull down
Chest	Chest press
Shoulders	Lateral raise
Arms	Biceps curl
	Triceps extension
Midsection	Crunches

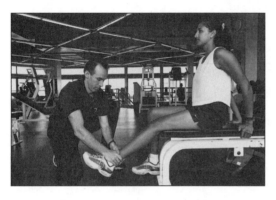

For the manual resistance leg extension, the spotter presses down on the lifter's ankle, while her upper leg is supported on the bench.

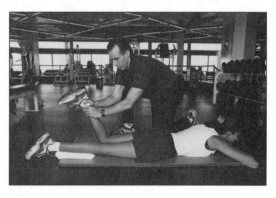

When performing a manual resistance leg curl, the lifter curls back as the spotter pushes against her.

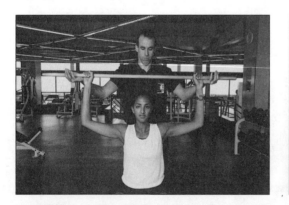

For the manual resistance lat pull down, the spotter pushes up on a broomstick as the lifter pulls down.

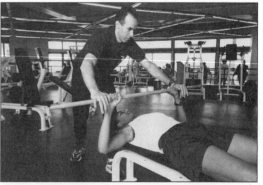

Here, the spotter pushes down on the broomstick as the lifter pushes up.

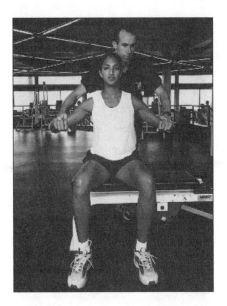

For the manual resistance lateral raise, the spotter presses down on the lifter's bent elbows.

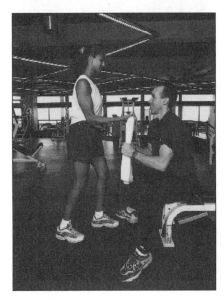

The spotter pulls down on a towel as the lifter curls it up.

Following the NSPA guidelines, here are the responsibilities of the *lifter:*

➤ Tension must be kept on the muscle.

➤ Must pause in contracted position.

➤ Must perform slow, smooth contractions.

➤ Must use full range of motion.

In the triceps extension, the spotter presses against the lifter's wrist.

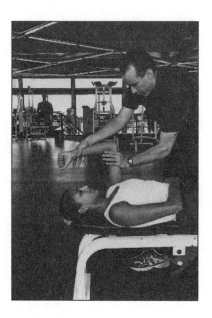

Here's the *spotter's* job:

➤ Must control smooth contractions and provide appropriate amount of resistance.

➤ Must control resistance so fatigue is reached within 10 to 15 repetitions.

➤ Must push in both the positive and the negative phase of the exercise.

When working as a spotter for the first time, err on the side of caution. Don't create too much resistance until you see what your partner can do. As the lifter, you have to give an honest effort on each rep; otherwise you won't get the results you're looking for.

Done properly, manual resistance exercises are a great, equipment-free way to get a challenging workout in a modest amount of time.

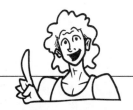

Workout Words

In manual resistance exercises, the person providing the resistance is referred to as the **spotter,** while the exercising half of the duo is the **lifter.**

Remember Calisthenics?

If all else fails, there's always good old-fashioned calisthenics (cals). No bands, no manual resistance, and certainly no machines or weights. Just you and your body weight. Cals are as pure a strength training as we know. They are tough and efficient and effective; maybe the best way you can use your valuable 15 minutes of exercise time.

Advantages of calisthenics:

➤ They can be done anywhere.

➤ They require virtually no equipment.

➤ They provide a very efficient workout.

Disadvantages of calisthenics:

➤ Resistance can't be varied.

➤ Limited number of exercises.

➤ Exercises may be too hard for some and too easy for others.

Let's talk about several of our favorite body weight exercises that you can do: push-ups (great for developing your chest, shoulders, and triceps), pull-ups and chin-ups (great exercises for your lats), and lunges (for your quads, hamstrings, and glutes).

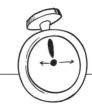

Short Cuts

If the lifter is much stronger than the spotter, try having the lifter hold light dumbbells during manual resistance exercises. The added weight can help make up for the disparity in strength. For instance, refer back to the lateral raises photo. If the spotter couldn't provide enough resistance, a pair five-pound dumbbells would give him some help.

Proper Push-Ups

Push-ups can be done with a variety of hand positions. Each hand position isolates a different part of your pecs. The standard, military variety uses a shoulder-width hand placement and works your pecs, shoulders, and triceps. Elevating your feet onto a chair, bed, or couch will shift the emphasis to the upper pecs and provide a little variety and far more difficulty. To place extra emphasis on your triceps, bring your hands together in a narrow position. To try the most difficult version of this push-up, form a triangle with your thumbs and index finger touching.

Once you've done your push-ups, it's time to work the opposing muscles.

Chin-Ups and Pull-Ups

These exercises against gravity remind us a bit of eating vegetables when you were a kid: You knew they were good for you, but you just couldn't bear to eat them. Similarly, these simple exercises are the toughest and most "cost effective" of any calisthenic exercise. For that reason, they are also two of the most neglected strength-training exercises. We know a handful of athletes who after adding pull-ups and/or chin-ups to their workout regimen made dramatic improvements in strength. In the

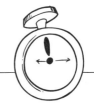

Short Cuts

If you want to do pull-ups and chin-ups at home, most sporting goods stores carry bars for just such a use. They're inexpensive and easily installed in a doorway.

beginning you will struggle to do even three or four good repetitions. Don't despair. If you stick with it and don't get discouraged, you will improve quickly and notice dramatic results.

Just as with push-ups, variations in hand positions provide some variety and shift the emphasis to different muscles. Regardless of hand position, you're using the muscles of your back on biceps exercises.

➤ The standard, military pull-up is performed with an overhand grip, with the hands slightly wider than shoulder width.

➤ The wide-grip pull-up—in case you can't figure it out—is a variation done with a wider grip. It's especially tough on your lats and the other muscles of your mid- and lower back.

➤ The chin-up is performed with a shoulder-width, underhand grip. It places extra emphasis on your biceps.

Learn to Lunge

Lunges are basically just one-legged squats. They work your quads, hamstrings, and glutes. You can use your body weight as resistance or, in a pinch, you can hold light dumbbells or anything else you have around (jugs of water work well). If you use weight, be sure to hold an equal amount in each hand. When you perform the lunge be sure to keep your torso upright and keep your front knee from passing forward of your big toe.

Note how Jonathan's back is straight and his knees are behind his toes as he finishes his lunge.

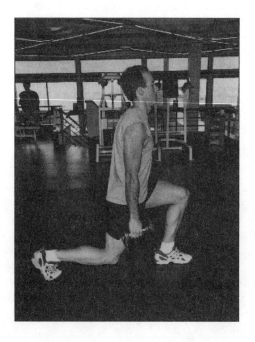

Creative Calisthenics

With just these three exercises and a couple of ab exercises, you can give your muscles a good workout. Try this routine:

> Lunges
>
> Push-ups (standard shoulder width hand placement)
>
> Push-ups (feet elevated, shoulder-width hand placement)
>
> Push-ups (narrow-width hand placement)
>
> Pull-ups (military grip)
>
> Pull-ups (wide grip)
>
> Chin-ups
>
> Crunches

Because you're moving your body weight (and not an adjustable stack of weights), you can't adjust the resistance—unless you have a spotter who can help give you a nudge on the way up. As a result, some people will do two or three pull-ups while others will be able to do 15 or 20. Your concern should be to gradually improve—don't worry about how many reps you can do. The key is maintaining good form and pushing yourself *to failure.*

Clearly, 15 minutes isn't a lot of time, but it is enough to give your muscles a good pump. Any of these routines—bands, manuals, or calisthenics—can be done in your office, living room, or hotel room. Remember that while 15 minutes isn't the same as a full workout in the gym that we describe in later chapters, it's far better than a day without exercise. Think about that the next time you're lounging on the couching watching ESPN.

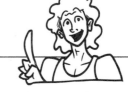

Workout Words

In gym speak, working **to failure** means to do as many repetitions as possible without sacrificing form or safety.

The Least You Need to Know

➤ While 15 minutes of strength training isn't enough time to enable you to be in the next Mr. or Ms. Olympia contest, it is enough time for you to get a basic foundation of strength.

➤ Though not our favorite choice, resistance bands can give you an effective workout when you have no alternative.

➤ Manuals can be a fun way to work out with a buddy and they are killer routines to boot.

➤ Forget all the fancy stuff; some of the best athletes sculpt their fabulous bodies by doing good old calisthenics.

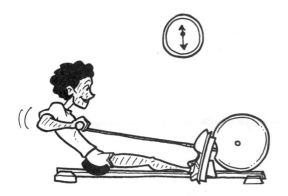

Chapter 11

The 30-Minute Cardio Workout

> **In This Chapter**
>
> ➤ Interval training gives your workout a boost
>
> ➤ Run your way to fitness
>
> ➤ Thirty-minute rides to get you fit and fast
>
> ➤ Cross-train for variety and health

If you want to get fit, a 30-minute cardio workout is a great place to start. It's not so long as to become tedious or intimidating, yet it's long enough to help you meet a variety of goals. Just as we stressed with the 15-minute workout (or any other for that matter), the key is to use your time well. Just pedaling aimlessly on the bike for half an hour isn't going to get you in shape, compared to a focused half-hour where you're concentrating on the task at hand. For that reason, nothing drives us battier than seeing someone sitting on the recumbent bike perusing the financial page oblivious to the reason they're on the bike in the first place—to actually break a sweat and get a good workout. Don't get us wrong, we're all for multitasking—hey, we're native New Yorkers after all—but a little focus can go a long way in making the difference between a fruitful workout and a near waste of time.

Here's a bit of math wizardry that you may need time to ponder: As we move from 15- to 30-minute workouts, there's twice as much time to work with. The extra 15 minutes means we don't have to find workouts that force you to jump rope like a hummingbird or climb stairs as if you're running for the last train home. Instead we can now have you do more conventional modes of exercise. Even with a warm-up and cooldown, half an hour is plenty of time to burn calories and improve your health.

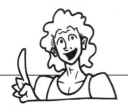

Workout Words

Interval training is the practice of alternating hard periods of exercise with easy periods to help you recover. Interval training is one of the most effective ways to increase your physiological capabilities.

Throughout this chapter we'll explain what interval workouts are and throw in a few other ideas such as cross-training and mini-triathlons. We'll give you workouts that you can do both at the gym or out in the real world.

Incorporate Intervals into Your Workout

Whether you're a seasoned athlete or a relative newcomer to exercise, we're big advocates of *interval training,* which means you alternate easy and hard efforts within the same workout. We especially like the format for short workouts because it's an efficient way to maximize the limited time so that you get the most out of it.

Steve Ilg, author of *The Winter Athlete* and a nationally known fitness trainer, said that the difference between serious and recreational athletes can be summarized in one word: *intervals.* To a certain extent he's correct. You should know, however, that intervals hurt. And the more you do, the more the discomfort. However, we believe that done properly (and in moderation), intervals will help you get the most fitness benefits from your workout. In essence, a 30-minute workout with intervals versus one without is, in fitness terms, nearly night and day. (Or at least night and twilight.)

Running Workouts

Running, which is perhaps the "purest" of all cardiovascular activities, (since it doesn't really require any equipment), is one of those "love" or "hate" activities. Why? Many people assume that when they go for a run, they have to push, push, push. Others try for half an hour when they're not fit enough to enjoy it. In fact, you may have learned the hard way that a 30-minute run can be a real challenge. In fact, if you can run for 30 minutes, you can count yourself among the proud minority—most people can't do half of that. Furthermore, if you can keep putting one foot in front of the other for half an hour, you might want to start thinking about trying your hand (or foot?) at a 5K (3.1-mile) race. Races are a great way to push yourself as well as get a taste of what your running community has to offer. You might find that while you don't "love" training, you really enjoy racing.

Here's an idea for a workout you can do in that time frame that will help you to become fitter and faster.

Most people who jog regularly tend to go out at the same pace most of the time. Furthermore, most of them hold that pace for the duration of their workout. This is fine if you're entirely happy with your performance, but it's not a great way to make improvements. If you fit into the "I'm doing okay, but I'd love to step it up a little" category, we have a suggestion for you.

Rather than simply going out for the same old run, try incorporating intervals into your workout. By picking up the pace for short periods throughout your run—say from one telephone pole to the next, or clock a minute or two on your watch—you help your body become acclimated to the increased stress. Eventually what was a hard interval becomes your cruising pace. When that happens, *voilà!* You're getting fitter.

Want a bit more structure to your running workout? Try this treadmill workout for a little extra oomph in your run:

1. Warm up with an easy five-minute jog.

2. Pick up the pace to a comfortable cruising pace for four minutes. The pace should be fast enough to get your heart rate to about 70 percent of your max.

3. Maintaining the same speed, add a 3 percent to 4 percent elevation *or* 0.5 miles per hour on the treadmill for one minute.

4. Repeat steps two and three, three more times.

5. Cool down with another easy five-minute jog.

Don't fret if you're running outdoors, and don't have a treadmill to keep track of things for you. If you're out on the road, try a *fartlek* workout. Here are a few examples:

➤ Every five minutes, sprint from one light pole to the next.

➤ If you're running on city streets, do a fast interval from one streetlight to the next every three minutes.

➤ A great way to gain strength if you're on hilly terrain is to take it easy on the flats and downhills and attack the inclines.

In other words, be creative with your workouts. When you're feeling good, let it rip. Challenge yourself a lot or just a bit; either way you'll find that adding a bit of intensity to your run will break up the monotony.

If you're not up for running, walking is a viable option. Use the same format as above—blocks of four moderate minutes and one hard minute—but substitute an incline on the treadmill in place of

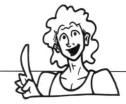

Workout Words

Don't get goofy with the gas jokes—**fartlek** is a Swedish word meaning "speed play." Fartlek workouts incorporate unstructured periods of bursts of speed. Rather than doing strictly structured intervals, you get to improvise and have some fun. Fartlek workouts are a form of interval training.

the faster run. Take long, forceful strides and pump your arms as you climb the hill. It'll still be a good cardio workout, yet you'll spare your body all the pounding and orthopedic stress of running.

Progress from Power Walking to Running

If you aspire to jog or run, but aren't able to pick up the pace quite yet, interval training can still be a useful strategy. By alternating walking and running, you can gradually get your body used to the faster speeds. For instance, let's suppose that you can comfortably walk at a pace of three miles per hour, but a moderate 5.5-mile-per-hour jog is too much for you to sustain for more than a few minutes.

Here's a six-week interval program that can help you progress from power walking to running. During weeks two to five, repeat the walk/jog pattern four times. Do each workout on three non-consecutive days for a week.

	Warm Up	Walk	Jog	Cool Down
Week 1	5 minutes	20 minutes		5 minutes
Week 2	5 minutes	4 minutes	1 minute	5 minutes
Week 3	5 minutes	3 minutes	2 minutes	5 minutes
Week 4	5 minutes	2 minutes	3 minutes	5 minutes
Week 5	5 minutes	1 minute	4 minutes	5 minutes
Week 6	5 minutes		20 minutes	5 minutes

Ride Workouts

There are few things that we enjoy more than a leisurely Sunday bicycle ride for a few hours on a beautiful spring day. Joe, who has taken the leisurely approach to a logical extreme, has ridden his bicycle from California to New York simply because it seemed like a good way to spend some of the summer. While Jonathan likes to tackle one state at a time, he, too, has spent countless hours in the saddle.

When you have the single-minded focus of a cross-country ride or want to become a strong competitive rider, logging big hours on your bike is the only way to travel. In fact, many of the guys that Jonathan races with don't feel it's worth slipping on Lycra shorts unless they're going to hit the pavement for an hour or more. Though we agree that you need to punch the clock hard and often if you want to ride with the big boys and girls, we're convinced that you can get a great ride in far less time as long as you have a focused workout.

For an indoor ride, we're partial to the Hill Profile program on the LifeCycle because it is a preprogrammed interval workout with a warm-up and cooldown. If you don't have access to a LifeCycle, fret not; there are plenty of other ways to make the most of your half-hour.

Stand and Deliver

Here's a revolutionary idea for all of you who complain that bicycle seats are uncomfortable: *don't use it!* Okay, we're not really advocating that you stand through an entire workout, but throwing in a few high-intensity intervals can really help you get the most out of a short workout. After five minutes of easy cycling at a high cadence (80 to 100 revolutions per minute) and low resistance, start to crank up the resistance. Try to get your heart rate to about 70 percent of your max. It should be challenging, but not hard. Then, once every five minutes spend one minute pedaling out of the saddle with the resistance cranked up.

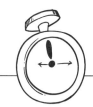

Imagine yourself grinding up a steep hill, keeping your cadence in the 50 to 60 revolutions-per-minute (rpm) range. Try to work hard enough to elevate your heart rate to around 85 percent of your max—or enough that your quadriceps are calling you nasty names. Repeat this five-minute sequence four times and finish things off with another five-minute spin. As you become fitter and your legs become acclimated to the workout, you can add the standing climbs more often. Progress from one every five minutes to one every four. Eventually try to alternate one minute standing and one minute seated. It's a great way work out your quads and cardiovascular system. We assure you that as your legs are quivering and you're sweating up a storm, you'll no longer have any concerns over whether a 30-minute workout is enough.

Short Cuts

Bicycle seats come in a variety of shapes and sizes. A comfortable model for one person is horribly painful for another, so take a few out for a test ride before making a purchase.

Turn on the Spin Cycle

Sit with a group of racing cyclists like Jonathan for more than five minutes and you're bound to hear them refer to their "spin." In cyclist's lingo, spinning is pedaling at a smooth, high cadence. Elite road and track cyclists often train at mind-boggling cadences in excess of 200 rpm—a pace that resembles chaotic eggbeaters. (Contrast that with the typical cadence of 50 to 60 rpm for casual commuters or 60 to 80 rpm for most exercisers in the gym.) While such astronomical spinning speeds are not necessary for regular fitness types, picking up the cadence is a great way to rev up your workout.

Rather than increasing the resistance and grinding at a low pedal cadence, try adding some spice to your workout with a faster spin for 20- to 30-second intervals.

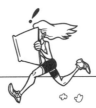

Info to Go

Jonathan was recently working with a client who complained that indoor cycling was so tedious that he'd started watching television in the gym to pass the time. While it can actually be inspiring to watch tapes of races such as the Tour de France, Jonathan suggested spicing up the workout by adding high-cadence spins during every other commercial. By incorporating these high-intensity intervals, Jonathan was sure that his client was getting a better cardiovascular workout while his client found that he was no longer bored, and in fact he enjoyed it.

Tri This

A few years back, the term *cross-training* became the buzzword within the fitness community. By alternating among several different sports such as cycling, running, and swimming, fitness enthusiasts found it much easier to avoid overuse injuries and boredom. Better yet, they were still able to get a great workout. Many athletes whose bodies had been subjected to countless hours of the same repetitive movement also found the benefits of cross-training were less time spent on the disabled list.

Indoor or Out

In 1997, Jonathan wanted to devise a challenging workout for some of the time-starved but ambitious cops at his fitness center. Many of them are excellent athletes who have a limited time to devote to working out. He also wanted to accommodate members who weren't in great shape yet. Jonathan figured a good way to put them to the test was to have a 30-minute "indoor triathlon"—a perfect example of cross-training at work. He laid out the following format:

Concept II rower	10 minutes
Stationary bike	10 minutes
Treadmill	10 minutes

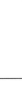

Workout Words

Cross-training is a training method that involves the use of a variety of exercises rather than one. For example, a runner might cross-train by using a cross-country ski machine or cycling once a week. Cross-training is an effective way to avoid muscle imbalances and overuse injuries.

The race consisted of 10 minutes on each machine with an oh-so-short one-minute transition between each.

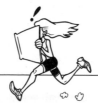

Info to Go

While the Hawaiian Ironman, which consists of a 2.4-mile swim, a 112-mile bike ride, and a 26.2-mile running marathon, is the best known triathlon, there are many other races of varying distances held throughout the world. The International or Olympic distance race is "only" a one-kilometer (.6-mile) swim, 40K (24.8-mile) ride, and 10K (6.2-mile) run. Shorter "sprint" distance races are also becoming more common. And there is an increasing number of multisport triathlons and quadathlons that include canoeing, kayaking, or mountain biking.

The beginners were able to handle the relatively user-friendly 30-minute format while the fitter, hard-charging athletes were wrecked after the surprisingly tough event. Combining the three modes used a variety of muscles and provided a more challenging workout than simply sitting on one piece of equipment for half an hour. More important, it also proved a point to the skeptics who thought it wasn't worth lacing on their sneakers for less than an hour.

Think Vertical

Each fall the local chapter of the American Lung Association holds a particularly cruel triathlon called the Vertical Challenge in Wilmington, Delaware, that can be duplicated in your gym. The race is a 5K (3.1-mile) run, 10K ride (6.2-mile), and then a quad-busting 22-story stair climb. Jonathan trained for this event almost exclusively in the gym, usually in 30-minute segments (or less).

Here's what our vertically challenged friend did:

Run	10 minutes
Ride	15 minutes
StairMaster	5 minutes

While we particularly like these two triathlon formats, there are countless other combinations you can use. Want a good low-impact workout? Try combining the recumbent bike, elliptical trainer, and Stairclimber. Need a little extra challenge for your upper body? How about the Concept II rower, NordicTrack cross-country skier, and the elliptical trainer? The point isn't so much what machines you cross-train on, but that you break the half-hour workout into manageable pieces that keep you stimulated and eager to push on. Another great thing about this format is that rotating among multiple machines not only helps reduce boredom, but you don't have to worry about your gym-mates looking over your shoulder because you're hogging one piece of equipment.

Remember that since you're in the gym to train, not to race, you don't need to go all out on these "triathlons." Aim to keep your heart rate in the 70 percent to 85 percent range.

The ideas we've presented in this chapter represent just a small fraction of the countless workouts that you can do in 30 minutes. Whether you use these specific workouts or not, the important thing to keep in mind is to stress quality over quantity. By incorporating intervals and ensuring that your heart rate remains within your training zone, you're sure to get the most out of your half-hour. Remember that a purposeful half-hour beats an unfocused hour or two of dilly-dallying any day.

The Least You Need to Know

➤ Thirty minutes of cardio can provide significant benefits.

➤ Intervals are an effective way to improve your fitness.

➤ You can run, walk, or ride your way to better health.

➤ A "minitriathlon" can make the time fly by and get you in great shape.

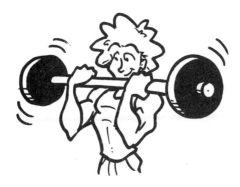

Chapter 12

The 30-Minute Strength-Training Workout

In This Chapter

➤ Have it all—in 30 minutes

➤ For upper-body fans

➤ Workouts that are heavy on the legs

➤ All-around sculpting for injury-free fitness

Thirty minutes—the time it takes to watch a sitcom—happens to be ample time to get a good, thorough, full-body workout in the gym. No, it's not enough to qualify for the Olympic weight-lifting team, but it's plenty to improve your health and fitness. In other words, train efficiently (and hard) for 30 minutes at a time and you will get stronger. In this chapter, we'll outline several training routines that you can cover in a half hour at the fitness center.

Upper-Body Emphasis

Here's a comprehensive 30-minute strength-training workout that will cover all your major muscle groups. Because we're using a limited amount of exercises, we've opted for lots of *multijoint exercises* to use as many muscles as possible in each exercise, rather than single-joint exercises. Each time you lift, remember to never sacrifice form just to squeeze out an extra rep. Perform each rep using slow controlled form and don't hold your breath.

Body Part	Exercise
Legs/hips	Leg press
Back	Lat pull down
	Upright rows
Chest	Chest press
	Dips
Shoulders	Shoulder press
Arms	Seated biceps curl
	Triceps push down
Midsection	Reverse crunch
	Crunch
	Back raise

Since we've introduced several new exercises, let's look at the proper form for each.

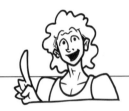

Workout Words

As the name suggests, **multi-joint exercises** work more than one joint at a time. In turn, they also use more than one muscle group and are therefore a good strategy when your lifting time is limited. Conversely, single-joint movements are best for isolating a particular muscle.

Leg Press

The leg-press machine is a great way to work lots of muscles (including the glutes, quads, and hamstrings) in just one exercise. Here's the lowdown on pressing the weights up:

1. Position yourself in the machine with your feet approximately shoulder width and your toes pointed out slightly.
2. Grasp the handles on either side of the seat.
3. Release the hand brake.
4. Lower the sled in a slow, controlled fashion for a count of three until your knees are at approximately a 90° angle.
5. Pause and press the weight back to the starting position as you exhale.

Leg Press Tips

Keep your back against the backrest at all times.

Keep your buttocks against the pad. Make sure you don't lose contact as you lower the weight.

Don't lock your knees at the top.

Keep your abdominals tight for stability.

All leg-press machines have a safety mechanism that prevents the weight from coming down too far. Make sure that the safety is set on the machine before you use it.

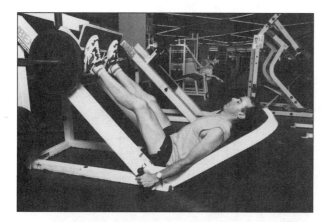

Remember not to lock your knees in the start/finish position of the leg press.

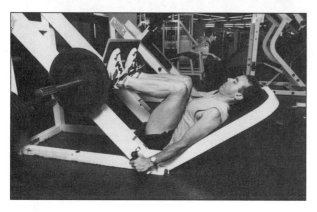

Bring the carriage down until your knees are at a right angle.

Lat Pull Down

Ever wonder how to get the great V-shape back that so many athletes have? The lat pull down is your ticket. Because strong lats are so vital to athletes in virtually every

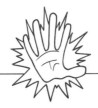

Stop Short

If you have shoulder impinge-ment syndrome or other shoulder problems, you should not do lat pull downs or upright rows until you're healthy again. When you resume, start really light and work your way up.

sport from swimming to squash, they're a staple of most every lifter's regimen. Here are the basics for the lat pull down:

1. Hold the bar with an overhand grip and your hands slightly wider than shoulder width apart.

2. Sit on the seat and make sure that your knees are securely tucked under the knee pads. (The knee pads are adjustable, so make sure your knees fit snugly under the pads.)

3. Pull the bar down to the base of your neck or your collarbone.

4. Pause and return the bar to the starting position.

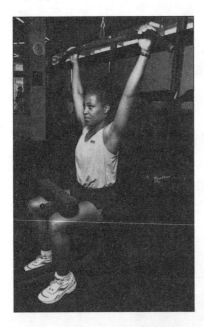

Make sure to get a good stretch in the start/finish position of the lat pull down.

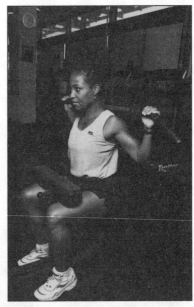

Note how Deidre's neck and back remain flat as she brings the bar down.

Lat Pull Down Tips

The lat pull down can be done with the bar pulled behind the neck or to the collarbone. If you use the behind-the-neck variation, be sure not to cock your head forward, since this makes you susceptible to muscle pulls.

Control the bar during the negative (or "easy") phase. Don't let the bar pull you up or out of your seat.

Keep your back flat as you pull the bar down.

Upright Row

The great thing about the upright row is that it works the trapezius, deltoids, and biceps all at one time. That's lots of muscle in just one exercise. Here's the rundown on the proper way to perform upright rows:

1. Stand with your feet shoulder width apart.
2. Hold the bar with a narrow, overhand grip (knuckles forward).
3. Pull the bar up to shoulder level.
4. Pause and lower the bar to the starting position in a controlled fashion.

Upright Row Tips

Keep the bar close to your body throughout the range of motion.

Keep your abs tight and your back flat.

Make sure that your elbows stay higher than your hands.

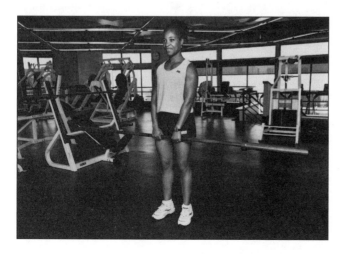

The arms should be fully extended in the start/ finish position for the upright row.

Note the high elbows and flat back at the top position.

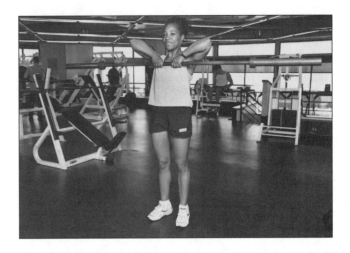

Chest/Bench Press

The bench press or chest press is *the* definitive upper-body exercise in most lifters' programs. Whether you use a machine, dumbbells, or a barbell, the chest press is a great way to work your pecs, deltoids, and triceps. If you're using free weights, be sure to use a spotter. Here's the deal on the free-weight bench press:

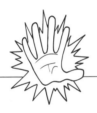

Stop Short

Holding your breath while lifting is known as the Valsalva maneuver. It's a common practice in the gym, but try strenuously to avoid it. Extreme fluctuations in blood pressure (and even fainting) can result from the Valsalva maneuver.

1. Lie on your back with your knees bent and your feet on the bench or flat on the floor. The floor gives you a little more stability, but make sure your legs are long enough to allow you to keep your back flat.

2. Hold the bar with a slightly wider-than-shoulder-width grip.

3. Lift the bar from the uprights (with the assistance of a spotter if necessary).

4. Slowly lower the bar to your chest (aim for the nipple line) while inhaling.

5. Pause at the bottom of the lift (at your chest) and then press the weight back to the starting position while exhaling.

Chest/Bench Press Tips

Never arch your back or lift your buttocks off the bench.

Don't hold your breath.

Keep your thumbs securely wrapped around the bar.

Don't lock your elbows at the extended position.

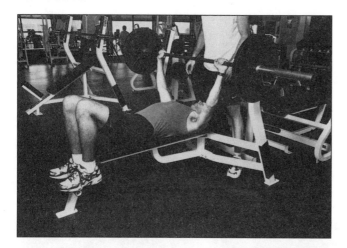

At the start/finish position of the bench press, your elbows should be bent ever so slightly.

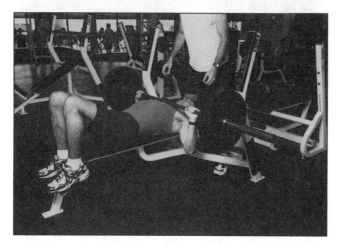

The bar should be slowly lowered until it lightly touches your chest.

Dips

Dips are also a great exercise to work your chest, shoulders, and triceps all at once. While it is one of the best multiple-body part exercises, there's one problem: Many people aren't strong enough to do even a few reps on their own. Luckily the Gravitron was invented a few years ago. The Gravitron, which sounds like a planet in an episode of *Superman,* allows the "dipper" to do dips (as well as pull-ups) with the assistance of a platform that helps push you up. You can program the machine to assist you a lot or hardly at all. Use it regularly and you'll be doing unassisted dips. Please note that the form remains the same whether you use your full body weight or a machine:

1. Position yourself between the handles, bend your knees, and hold yourself up by keeping your elbows straight. If you're using a Gravitron or similar machine, keep your feet flat on the platform.

2. Slowly bend your elbows and lower your body until your upper arms are parallel to the ground.

3. Return to the starting position.

Dips Tips

Don't arch your back or throw your head into the exercise.

Keep your chest up.

Don't lock your elbows at the top of the movement.

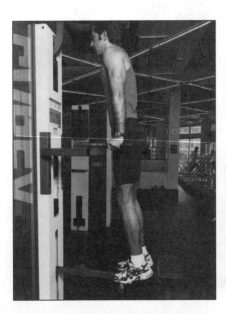

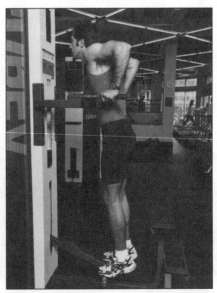

In the start/finish position of the dip, your torso should be straight and your elbows slightly bent.

Lower yourself until your upper arms are parallel to the floor.

Shoulder Press

The shoulder press—sometimes known as the military press—is a great way to blast your deltoids and help build broad shoulders. Much like the chest press, you can effectively do the exercise using a machine, barbell, or dumbbells. Here's the drill for the dumbbell military press (get it?):

1. Sit on a bench with a dumbbell in each hand. Be sure to sit up straight and use a bench with a backrest if available.

2. Raise the dumbbells with your palms facing inward.

3. Hold them at a right angle with the dumbbells by your shoulders.

4. Slowly raise your arms and bring the dumbbells together.

5. Slowly lower the dumbbells to the starting position.

6. Concentrate on your breathing, especially as you near failure.

Shoulder Press Tips

Never arch your back.

Don't bang the dumbbells together.

Keep your abs tight and your head and neck straight.

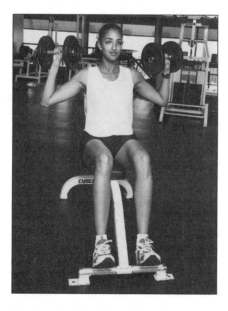

In the start/finish position, the dumbbells should be just above shoulder level.

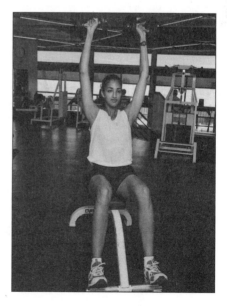

Extend until your elbows are almost straight.

Seated Biceps Curl

At last count, there were no fewer than 5,000 exercises you could do for your biceps (and many folks in the gym do all of them). We particularly like the seated biceps curl because it's a little harder to cheat on your form than with other biceps exercises. Here are the basics:

1. Sit with a dumbbell in each hand and your palms facing inward.

2. Slowly bend your elbows, twisting your wrists and bringing your palms up as you do.

3. Continue to curl the weight up until the dumbbells near your shoulders. (Don't bring them all the way up.)

4. Slowly lower the weight, twisting your wrists back to the starting position.

Biceps Curl Tips

Keep your elbows in close against your body.

Don't arch your back or hold your breath.

Avoid shrugging your shoulders as you curl the weight.

In other words, choose a weight that you don't have to "cheat" to lift the last few repetitions of each set.

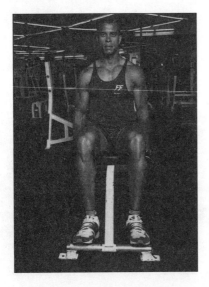 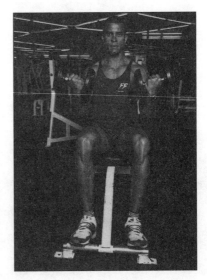

In the start/finish position, the dumbbells should be at your sides with your palms inward.

As you curl the weight up to the midrange position, keep your elbows tucked in.

Triceps Push Down

Like biceps exercises, there are countless options to choose from when it comes time to working your triceps, those three muscles at the rear of your upper arm. We'll show you a few more later, but right now let's stick with our favorite: the triceps push down:

1. Hold the push-down bar on a pulley of a lat pull-down or cable cross machine with your wrists straight and your elbows bent at about 90° and close to your sides.

2. Slowly straighten your elbows.

3. Return to the starting position in a slow, controlled manner.

Triceps Push-Down Tips

Don't lean forward as you do the exercise—that makes it easier, not more effective.

Keep your abs tight and your back straight.

Don't let your elbows drift up.

Keep your head neutral, not facing up, down, or to the sides.

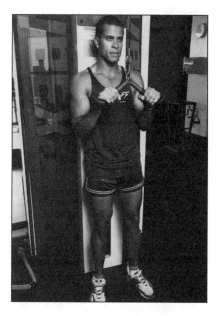

At the start, your elbows should be bent and tucked in at your sides.

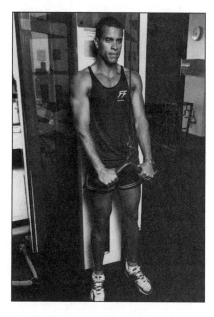

At the bottom of the push-down motion, stop just short of locking your elbows and keep them close at your sides.

143

Back Raise

It's important to maintain a balance between your opposing muscles: biceps and triceps, quadriceps and hamstrings, for example. Why? So you don't risk injury as one muscle group becomes stronger than its opposite. While most people make sure to work their abdominal muscles, often they neglect the muscle of the lower back. The best way to work the muscles that oppose your abs are back raises.

The back raise can be done on a machine as well as on specially designed benches that are becoming more common in the gym. If all else fails, you can do it on a mat by simply lying on your stomach with your hands behind your back while slowly and gently using your lower back muscles to lift your head and chest off the mat. We prefer the machine because it allows you to vary the resistance and gives you a fuller range of motion. Here are the basics:

1. Begin in the forward position.

2. Strap yourself in using the seat belt that is standard on most machines.

3. Using your lower back muscles, press back against the pad.

4. Pause at the fully extended position.

5. Slowly return to the starting position.

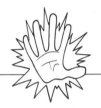

Stop Short

Neglecting to train opposing muscle groups can lead to muscle imbalances and injuries. For instance, if you strengthen your quadriceps, you should be sure to work on your hamstrings as well.

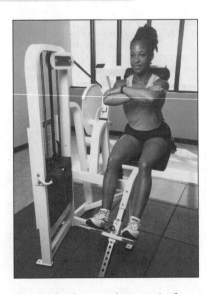

For the back extension, you're bent forward at the waist for the start/ finish position.

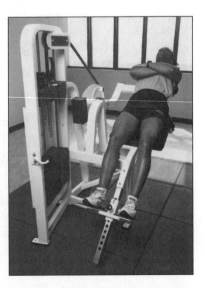

As you perform the back extension, slowly move backward until your back is flat.

Back Raise Tips

Push with your lower back muscles, not your legs.

Always wear the seat belt—it will help minimize cheating.

Don't throw your head back or turn your head.

Lower-Body Emphasis

While we like the routine listed above, no one will ever call it too heavy on leg exercises. We love the leg-press machine because it works so many muscles. In addition, the inclusion of a few more exercises in the following routine will allow you to build stronger, buffer legs.

Body Part	Exercise
Legs/hips	Leg press
	Leg curl
	Leg extension
Back	Lat pull down
Chest	Chest press
Shoulders	Shoulder press
Arms	Seated biceps curl
	Triceps push down
Midsection	Reverse crunch
	Crunch
	Back raise

In this routine we've removed a couple of upper-body exercises (upright rows and dips) and added leg curls and leg extensions. It still leaves plenty of upper-body exercises, but the inclusion of the extra leg exercises balances things out.

Here's a rundown on the proper form for the two new exercises.

Leg Curl

The leg curl is the best exercise to isolate your hamstrings (the large muscles located on the back of your thighs). The proper form is as follows:

1. Lie face down on the machine and place your lower legs underneath the rollers.

2. Position yourself so that your kneecaps are just off of the edge of the pad.

3. Grasp the handles on either side of the machine.

4. Slowly bend your knees and curl the weight up toward your buttocks.

5. Pause at the top of the movement and slowly return to the starting position.

Leg Curl Tips

Don't arch your back or pick your pelvis up off the machine.

Don't turn your head. Instead rest your forehead on the machine. (A towel comes in handy if you need to wipe off the machine.)

Make sure that you curl until you reach an angle of at least 90°.

In the start/finish position for the leg curl, there is a slight bend in the knees.

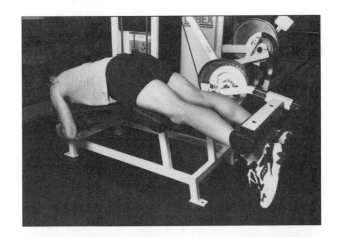

Your hamstrings help you bend your knees. Stop at about a 90° angle.

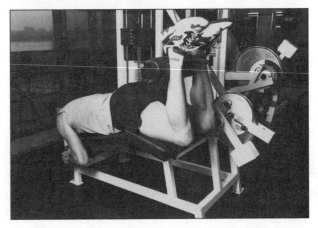

Leg Extension

The leg extension (coincidentally, performed on the leg extension machine) is the definitive exercise to work the quadriceps. As always, focus on good form, since trying to move too much weight leaves you susceptible to injury. Here's what you need to know:

1. Sit with your back against the pad with the bottom of your shins behind the leg pad.
2. Hold the handles on either side of the seat.
3. Slowly raise the pad until your legs are almost straight.
4. Pause and then slowly lower the weight to the starting position.

Leg Extension Tips

Don't swing the weight.

Don't lock your knees at the extended position.

Keep your back against the pad and your butt in the seat.

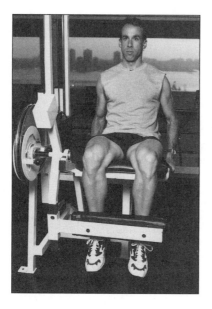

The start/finish position of the leg extension is as easy as sitting down.

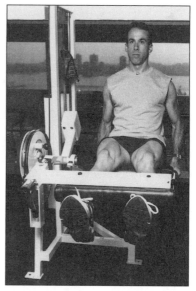

In the middle position, you should be sure to remain planted in the seat and keep a slight bend in your knees.

In future chapters, we'll introduce more exercises and ideas about how to break up your workouts if you have extra time to spend in the gym. In the meantime, we hope we've convinced you that 30 minutes is plenty of time for a good strength workout. If you don't believe us, try it for a few weeks and see for yourself.

The Least You Need to Know

➤ Thirty minutes can give you legitimate strength gains.

➤ By performing multijoint exercises, you work several muscles simultaneously, saving time and getting strong in the meantime.

➤ Work all opposing muscle groups—biceps and triceps, quadriceps and hamstrings—to avoid muscle imbalance injuries.

Part 4

The Workouts: 45 Minutes to 60 Minutes

While we firmly believe that 30 well-planned minutes a day are enough to help whip you into shape, the luxury of a little more time can certainly come in handy. This part looks at what you can do in 45 to 60 minutes.

We give you a rundown of how to get a full workout in 45 minutes, complete with stretching, cardio, and strength training. Then we move up to a full hour and outline plans for a 60-minute workout that addresses your flexibility, strength, and cardiovascular needs. In addition, we'll suggest workouts for the recreational athlete to help improve your game without taking you away from it for too long.

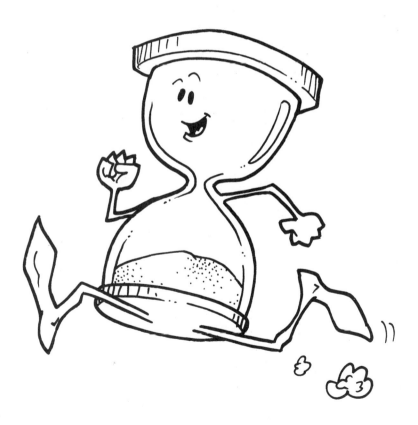

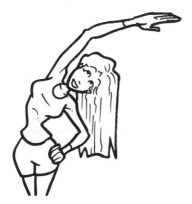

Chapter 13

The 45-Minute Workout

In This Chapter

➤ The perils of not warming up or cooling down

➤ Getting in and getting out—how to cover all the bases in 45 minutes

➤ Covering all the bases—cardio, strength, and stretching

➤ A workout routine to follow

We hope that by now we've convinced you that the key to getting in shape isn't how long you work out, but how hard and how often. You want to be fit? You want to actualize the body that you've pictured in your mind's eye? Frequency, desire, and intensity are your biggest allies—not the ability to block out huge chunks of time. (Combine desire and intensity with big hours and you've got the makings of an Ironman triathlete.) If you supply the discipline to get to the gym and follow our guidelines, we'll help you realize your fitness dream.

Once we've got you in the gym you're only halfway there. The next step is to eliminate the "nonessential" parts of your routine: taking too long between sets, talking to Harry about his weekend, and more. Finally, we'll give you a variety of workouts that can be done in as little as a few minutes at your desk to one hour at the gym. All these workouts are high on efficiency. The common denominator is they'll all help improve your fitness.

The Breakdown

You'll notice that now that we've graduated all the way up to a luxurious 45 minutes, we're outlining workouts that address all the major fitness issues in one session: flexibility, strength, and cardiovascular endurance. No, three-quarters of an hour is not exactly a lot of time in which to cover all these aspects, but with some focus and determination, you can get it done.

Here's a thumbnail sketch of how to break down your 45-minute workout:

➤ Warm-up (5 minutes)

➤ Cardiovascular (15 minutes)

➤ Cooldown (5 minutes)

➤ Strength training (15 minutes)

➤ Stretch (5 minutes)

With a relatively modest 15 minutes each for strength training and cardio, you can't expect miracles, but done right, you can expect a productive workout.

Let's take a closer look at the components that we want you to do.

Get Warm

We constantly hear people say, "I'm pressed for time, can't I skip the warm-up?" as if not warming up is like skipping the appetizer and jumping to the main course. People often offer creative reasons why it's a waste of time, including, "I'm naturally limber," or, "I work out regularly and usually do it." Our answer for the last 9,743 times is, "No!"

Here's why. Just as you'd never see a runner show up for a 10K road race, pull off his or her sweats, and tear off, the warm-up before your workout serves several important physiological purposes. (Actually, the warm-up is part of your workout; people think of it as something separate.)

Here's how it works: As the name implies, your warm-up literally raises your body temperature. Without "priming the pump," your body is less efficient at transferring oxygen from your blood to the working muscles. Put another way, warm up properly and your workout will be easier and better. Better still, this oft-neglected part of workout increases blood flow to your muscles, which lubricates your joints; which greatly decreases your risk of injury when you run, bike,

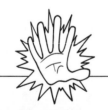

Stop Short

While it's tempting to save time by skipping your warm-up, it's also a really bad idea. The warm-up not only makes your workout safer, it makes it more effective as well.

swim, or lift. Skip the warm-up and the odds of pulling a muscle go way up along with the number of workouts you'll have to miss.

Okay, you're saying, I'm completely ready to lubricate my joints; what should I do for a warm-up? Think of your old high school gym teacher who had you do a couple of quick toe touches and jumping jacks—and do the exact opposite. Your warm-up should consist of a light workout on a piece of cardiovascular equipment such as a stationary bike, rowing machine, or cross-country ski machine.

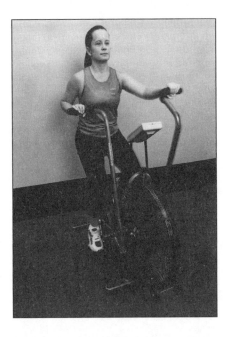

Schwinn Air Dyne bike. This is one of our favorites because you get to set the pace and it uses both your arms and your legs.

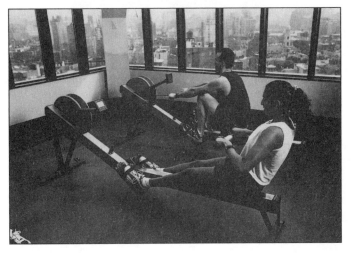

Concept II rower. Designed for rowers by rowers, this incredibly efficient piece of exercise equipment does much the same as the Air Dyne.

The cross-country ski machine is another great warm-up that uses both your upper body and your lower body.

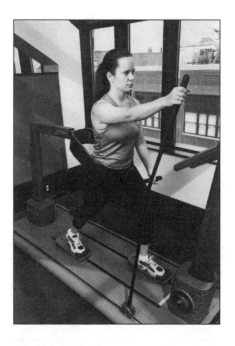

Though we prefer machines that use both your upper and your lower body, a treadmill or bike will do just fine. When you warm up, your heart rate should be about 50 percent of your max, or hard enough to get you to break just a light sweat. (In Chapter 5, "Aerobics," we laid out guidelines to help you figure out your training heart rate. The best way to figure out your absolute maximum is to get chased by a bear; however, if you don't outrun the beast the information is useless.)

Cardiovascular Workouts

Once you warm up you're ready to slide directly to your cardiovascular workout. Since time is limited, our aim is to make each cardio session pay ample dividends. That doesn't mean we're going to have you running stadium steps until you toss your cookies. (Although if you live near a stadium we're happy to oblige with some heart-stomping stair climbing.) On the other hand, we're here to work out, not have a cup of tea. Twenty to 30 minutes is enough only if you do it right. We all know people who log conspicuous cardiovascular (CV) time on a stationary bike who turn the pages of the magazine more vigorously than they're turning the pedals. That's okay if you're eager not to sweat on what you're reading, but it's not going to get you any fitter. (We're all for literacy, but not during your valuable fitness time.) Remember, you don't have to flog yourself silly to get a good workout, but staying awake does help.

In Chapter 5 we explained that you receive the greatest benefit from your cardiovascular exercise if you train within specific target heart-rate zones. As a rule, training between 60 percent and 85 percent of your maximum heart rate is your best bet for improving your cardiovascular fitness. When your time is limited, we prefer you train at the high end of that zone—75 percent to 85 percent—for a substantial part of your workout time. The good news is that at this intensity you'll burn more calories than at a lower intensity. The bad news is that if you're not used to working out at this pace, it will feel difficult. Most people, even competitive athletes, find it difficult to sustain 85 percent effort for much more than half an hour. Nevertheless, it's an ideal level of exertion to improve your cardiovascular system.

Here are a few of our favorite indoor cardio workouts to do when you've got roughly 15 minutes to spend.

➤ **The Lifecycle hill profile.** The Lifecycle is still the most frequently found stationary bike in health clubs around the country. One of the standard Lifecycle programs is the "hill profile," which simulates hill climbing. The increased resistance provides a form of *"interval training,"* which is one of the most effective ways of improving your cardiovascular fitness. Lifecycles can be set for level 1 through 12. (One is easy; 12 is a grunt-fest.) Find one where the last couple of hills are challenging, but don't require an all-out effort.

➤ **The StairMaster Lunar Landing program.** Actually, the StairMaster has several programs that we like, but this is one of our favorites. As with the Lifecycle, it has a built-in warm-up and cooldown and variable levels to suit your fitness level.

➤ **Concept II (C2) rower intervals.** One of the differences between the Concept II and most other pieces of cardiovascular gym equipment is that it requires you to set the pace. Unlike a treadmill where you set the speed and had better keep up or else (picture George Jetson with Astro on a runaway treadmill), the C2 is at your command. After a five-minute warm-up, try alternating intervals of one hard minute with one easy minute for 10 minutes, followed by an easy five-minute cooldown. Concentrate on good form: focus on the muscles of your legs, rather than overstressing your back and arms.

Workout Words

Interval training is working out at varying levels of high and low intensity, such as running on the treadmill at 6.5 miles per hour for 5 minutes followed by running at 5 miles per hour for 10 minutes.

Cooldown

Ever notice that at the end of a marathon the volunteers urge the weary runners to continue walking around? If those wasted and wobbly runners who just ran 26.2 miles can tough it out and cool down for a few minutes, so can you. We see it all the time: people rushing through a workout and skipping their cooldown. Like the warm-up, the cooldown is an important part of a safe workout, maybe even more so. By the end of your cardiovascular workout, you've increased your heart rate, body temperature, and blood pressure significantly. In addition, your blood supply has been shifted to the working muscles (usually your legs). If you stop your workout abruptly, your blood will stay down in those muscles, which, in extreme cases, can lead to dizziness or even passing out.

Five minutes or so of easy exercise (about 30 percent to 50 percent of the speed and intensity) on the cardiovascular equipment you were using last should do the trick. For most people, cooling down until their heart rate is below 100 beats per minute is a good guideline.

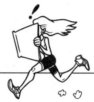

Info to Go

We'll spare you the gory details, but we know of several cases of people drowning after skipping a cooldown and going straight to a whirlpool where they lost consciousness. While this sounds too dramatic to be of real concern, in grad school one of Jonathan's classmates devised a twisted experiment designed to shed some light on the dangers of skipping a cooldown. The human guinea pigs had the "pleasure" of jumping into a whirlpool directly after a hard workout. Without a cooldown, body temperatures and blood pressures were astronomically high, even in healthy 20-year-old students.

Stretching

In Chapter 9, "The 15-Minute Workout," we talked about the importance of stretching. While we're obviously big stretch fans, we cringe when we watch someone walk into the gym and immediately start stretching like a platoon of West Point cadets. While we appreciate their good intentions, this approach often leads to pulled muscles and assorted other bad physical sensations. Unless you've jogged to the gym, warm up first. In other words, stretching cold muscles is a strict no go. Stretch after you've done your warm-up or at the end of your workout and your body will thank you. As we said earlier, don't stretch to the point of pain; hold the stretch for 20 to 30 seconds and don't bounce.

Here's a good basic stretching routine you can follow that covers most of your major muscle groups and won't take all day:

❏ Groin stretch

❏ Hip stretch

❏ Seated hamstring stretch

❏ Quadriceps stretch

❏ Standing calf stretch

Refer back to Chapter 7, "Start with Stretching," for a how-to guide to these stretches.

Strength Training

Often when we tell people that they can make serious strength-training gains in as little as 15 minutes, they look puzzled and say, "What can I do in such a miniscule amount of time?" Our answer? Plenty.

Jonathan, a champion number cruncher, figures it out like this: A set of 10 reps at 6 seconds per rep should take about a minute. A minute recovery between sets leaves you time for eight exercises. That may not sound like much, but it's enough to let you hit all your major muscle groups once. The minimal recovery between sets is probably far less than you're used to, so coupled with some hard sets, you're likely to find it more challenging than you might expect.

Here are two eight-set routines you can do, depending on what muscles you want to emphasize. In both cases, you'll progress from larger to smaller muscles, one stressing your lower body muscles and the other concentrating above your waist. Either scenario will hit all your major muscle groups.

Leg Emphasis

❏ Leg press	❏ Lat pull down
❏ Leg extension	❏ Shoulder press
❏ Leg curl	❏ Reverse crunch
❏ Chest press	❏ Crunch

Upper-Body Emphasis

❏ Leg press	❏ Upright row
❏ Lat pull down	❏ Shoulder press
❏ Chest press	❏ Reverse crunch
❏ Row	❏ Crunch

Remember, never lift using the same muscles on consecutive days. So if you did one of these routines on, say, Monday, don't do it again until Wednesday. If you really want to work out on Tuesday, plug in some extra cardio work.

The Least You Need to Know

➤ Time constraints don't excuse you from the most important aspects of your workout: the warm-up, stretching, and the cooldown.

➤ Forty-five minutes is plenty of time to get an efficient and effective workout.

➤ To emphasize lower or upper-body strengthening, follow the routines we've outlined for you.

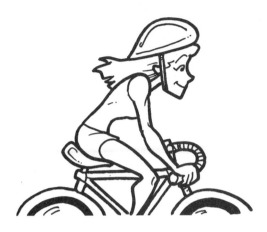

Chapter 14

The 45-Minute Cardio Workout

In This Chapter

➤ Getting the most out of 45 minutes of cardio

➤ Great ideas for running and riding

➤ Rowing is one of the best ways to get in shape

➤ No-impact fitness

Now that we've worked out all the way up to 45 minutes worth of cardiovascular exercise, there's finally some room to work with—no more rushing to get in and out before Judge Judy renders her verdict. As always, be sure to heed our warnings from the previous chapter and get good and warmed up before you get fully into the swing of things, and give yourself five minutes at the end to cool down.

Depending on your size and the intensity of your workout, you can figure on burning anywhere between 350 and 600 calories in three-quarters of an hour of sweating. While that's still not enough to justify bingeing on Twinkies, consistently doing 45-minute workouts three or four times a week is enough to make a significant contribution to weight loss if that's your goal. In this chapter we'll provide you with a variety of ideas of how to use that time to your greatest benefit.

Fun Running

While many runners would rather run naked through a bad neighborhood during a blizzard than run on a treadmill, we actually like them. If you use them correctly, treadmills can be invaluable training tools. Think about it: no getting stuck at traffic lights, no negotiating through puddles, potholes, and people—just smooth, focused running.

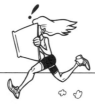

Info to Go

In fact, Jonathan's friend Christopher Bergland, a top East Coast triathlete, has trained for an Ironman triathlon and even a double Ironman (yes, it's what you think) exclusively on a treadmill. (For the record, an Ironman triathlon consists of a 2.4 mile swim followed by a 112 mile bike leg and a 26.2 mile run. A double Ironman is 4.8, 224, and 52.4 and takes the winner about 24 hours.) Rest assured, we're not going to suggest that you prepare for anything quite so crazy as an Ironman triathlon in 45 minutes a day, but we do feel strongly that treadmills are a great training tool.

One of the really neat things about a treadmill is that it lets you create implausible courses. (Though some runners we know—in defiance of the immutable laws of physics—would tell you that they have run an out-and-back course that's uphill in both directions, we remain skeptical.)

Here's an indoor hill workout that we especially like:

1. The workout begins innocently enough, with a five-minute warm-up at a comfortable pace, gradually increasing the speed until you reach about 65 percent of your max heart rate.

2. Hold that pace for another five minutes. If you're an experienced runner, this pace will feel very easy—the kind of pace you can hold all day. After the first 10 minutes, the fun begins with the following series of hills:

   ➤ 3 minutes at 1 percent elevation.

   ➤ 3 minutes flat.

   ➤ 3 minutes at 2 percent elevation.

   ➤ 3 minutes flat.

   ➤ 3 minutes at 3 percent elevation.

   ➤ 3 minutes flat.

➤ 3 minutes at 4 percent elevation.

➤ 3 minutes flat.

➤ 3 minutes at 5 percent elevation.

➤ 3 minutes flat.

3. Finish up with an easy five-minute walk to cool down.

Keep the speed constant throughout the workout— the elevation changes are what provide the challenge. Hills are a great way to break up the monotony of a workout as well as improve your running.

As we've mentioned, though interval training can be very rewarding for your body, it is also very taxing. Try it once or twice a week, alternating with easier, more moderately and steadily paced workouts to avoid the perils of *overtraining*. Overtraining can lead to illness and injury as well as a disturbance in sleep patterns.

As we said, away from the gym you will obviously be hard-pressed to find a course that allows you to duplicate the workout that's outlined above. Despite the limitations of the real world, you can still use hills to help get a great workout.

Find a hill that's about a quarter of a mile long with a moderate grade and get ready to burn some calories. Here's the drill for training on hills:

1. Warm up with an easy jog for five minutes.

2. Pick up the pace to about 65 percent to 70 percent max heart rate for another five minutes.

3. Run up the hill, running a hard, but controlled pace. Keep your strides long and your head up. Pace yourself and aim to finish as fast as you start.

4. Jog easily down the hill.

5. Repeat steps three and four as many times as possible in 30 minutes.

6. Cool down with an easy jog/walk on level ground for five minutes.

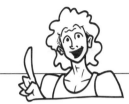

Workout Words

Overtraining occurs when you work out excessively, without sufficient recovery. You can avoid overtraining by taking at least one day off from exercise per week, and by avoiding consecutive days of hard workouts.

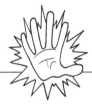

Stop Short

If you're not wearing a heart-rate monitor and can't be bothered to take your own pulse, judge your pace by how you feel. A good, albeit imperfect, barometer that's often used is the "talk test." For the "comfortable" sections, you should be able to speak a full sentence or two without huffing and puffing and having to catch your breath between words.

Either of the running workouts we've described is challenging, so don't try them more than once or twice a week. Use the other days for more moderately paced, steady workouts.

Ride Like the Wind

Whether you're out on the road or on a Lifecycle or other indoor bike, you can get a great workout in 45 minutes. Bikes are great for interval training because you can easily change the intensity—whether it's by shifting gears or pedaling faster on the road, or adjusting the resistance in the indoor bike.

If you're on the road, you can obviously use hills for your higher-intensity intervals during your ride. Don't fret if the terrain is flat—there are still other ways to work hard. Here's an old cyclists' trick: Find a section with a headwind and then shift into a harder gear rather than an easier one. You'll find that your cadence (revolutions per minute) decreases because of the combination of larger gear and headwind, and it feels similar to riding a hill.

In the gym, it's obviously a little easier to manipulate the "course" that you ride. Most electronic bikes have hill programs built in, and you can always use a spinning bike even when no class is in session. By increasing the resistance for two to three minutes at a time and grinding it out at a lower pedaling rate, you can simulate hills and give your ride some extra oomph.

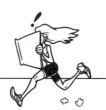

Info to Go

Back in 1981, the original Concept II Indoor Rower was introduced. At first it was a fairly primitive design, using a bicycle wheel where the nice, smooth fan on the current model is. It was made by and for competitive rowers, but it soon became a staple in fitness centers throughout the world.

Go Row

We've already mentioned several times that we think very highly of the Concept II (C2) rower. It uses the muscles of your upper and lower body, as well as your midsection, and you can't beat it for a cardiovascular workout.

Today hundreds of thousands of fitness enthusiasts use them, and in 1999, more than 15,000 people participated in races using the C2. In fact, Joe competed in a C2 race affectionately known as the "Valentine's Day Massacre" back in 1996 for an article he was writing for *The New York Times*. With a little coaching from Jonathan (mostly "go faster, Joe"), Joe even managed to win his division that day.

If you're just getting started with the C2, 10 or 15 minutes will be plenty. Since you're using muscles in a way that they're probably not used to, trying to do more right off the bat is inviting injury. Once you become a C2 veteran, you can try several longer workouts that we like. Here's one of our favorites:

1. Warm up at a gradually increasing pace for five minutes.

2. Pull at a moderate pace for five minutes; aim for 70 percent max heart rate.

3. One hard minute; aim for 85 percent of max heart rate. (Watch the strokes per minute and output readings on the monitor.) Then do the following intervals:

   ➤ Five minutes—easy.

   ➤ Two minutes—hard.

   ➤ Five minutes—easy.

   ➤ Three minutes—hard.

   ➤ Five minutes—moderate.

   ➤ Four minutes—hard.

   ➤ Five minutes—moderate.

4. Cool down at an easy pace for five minutes.

This workout is yet another example of interval training. The gradually increasing duration of the harder intervals will make the last one both challenging and physiologically rewarding.

One final note about the rowing machine. Don't be fooled by the implausibly broad backs and impressively muscular arms that you see on competitive rowers. While the rowing machine certainly uses far more upper-body muscle than most other cardio machines, the majority of your power should still come from your legs. Be sure to keep your back flat and your arms straight until you've fully extended your legs, otherwise you'll sacrifice your power output.

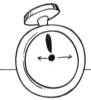

Short Cuts

If you're the competitive type, the Concept II even has online rankings that allow you to submit your results in events ranging from 500 meters (figure on a couple of minutes) to 26.2 miles (don't plan on getting out of the seat for a few hours). C2 also has a "million meter club" for those who accumulate a lot of rowing time.

No-Impact Workouts

One of the main complaints that we hear from recreational and competitive athletes alike is that their bodies take a pounding. Running and, to a lesser extent, cycling and other activities can each take their toll on your musculoskeletal system. Luckily there are some gentler, yet equally effective, pieces of equipment in the gym. Let's take a look at a couple of the most popular ones.

Elliptical Trainers

Elliptical trainers, also known as cross-trainers, are fast becoming one of the most popular pieces of equipment in gyms around the country. Introduced just a few years

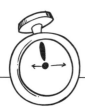

Short Cuts

There are lots of fun things you can do with an elliptical trainer—many have adjustable inclines and preprogrammed courses that create a variety of interval schemes. One feature that many people neglect is that most elliptical trainers can go backward. By reversing your stride every few minutes you can give your muscles a different feel for a few minutes at a time, while keeping your heart rate elevated. Try it for a change of pace.

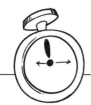

Short Cuts

The drawback to ski machines is that it requires time to learn. Because it uses all four limbs, unless you're an experienced cross-country skier (or a drummer), expect a couple of workouts to get fully into the swing of things. The best way to use the NordicTrack is by starting with just your legs and incorporating the arms once the lower-body movement becomes comfortable.

ago, they're now widely used by runners who want a no-impact workout. They're easy to use and quite gentle on the joints.

In 1998, when Jonathan's friend Grace DePompo, a top New York City runner and ten-time winner of New York's annual Police Fire Run, injured her back, she was unable to run for several months. For a competitive runner of her caliber, being put on the shelf for an extended period is worse than having bamboo stuck under her fingernails while listening to a Marilyn Manson album. In an effort to make lemonade out of the lemons that had been thrust upon her, Grace took to the elliptical trainer. She found that she was able to tolerate it because it didn't cause nearly as much orthopedic stress as pounding the pavement. By working out religiously on the elliptical machine until her back healed, Grace was able to return to top form far quicker than she ever anticipated and even chalk up her eleventh win in the Police Fire race.

In case you think the elliptical is just another passing fitness fad, you'll be comforted to know that studies have shown that when exercisers set their own pace, heart rate and oxygen consumption (two of the best indicators of the intensity of your workout) on the elliptical and a treadmill are comparable. That confirms for us physiologist types that the elliptical may be a smart way for runners to cross-train without the impact of running. Because the elliptical is so easy on the joints, many people find that a 45-minute workout on one leaves them much less achy or tired than a similar running workout, making it a great alternative to your usual gym routine.

Ski Cross-Country Indoors

The NordicTrack or some other cross-country ski simulator is another great way to get a no-impact workout that spares your joints, yet provides a fine cardiovascular and calorie-burning workout. By working your arms and legs, it involves most of your body's major muscle groups. We particularly like it once or twice a week if you've been working out hard and need to give your body a bit of a break. We find it's best suited for steady workouts, rather than intervals, so try it on a day after a challenging interval or hill workout.

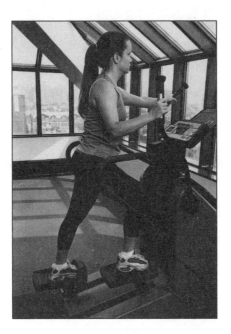

The elliptical trainer provides a great, impact-free cardiovascular workout.

The Nordic Track has independent resistance controls for the arms and legs, so you can place extra emphasis on either, while still getting the cardiovascular benefit. Unlike many other machines in the gym that have elaborate electronic monitors and programs, the NordicTrack is totally under your control. You set the pace, rather than having it set for you as on a treadmill. While this makes it impossible to set specific workouts, it does allow you to do most anything you want.

As you can see, 45 minutes is more than enough time to help you toward your goal of weight loss, cardiovascular fitness, and improved sports performance. The use of a variety of equipment and both interval and steadily paced workouts ensures that you get the most out of your exercise. If you've fallen into a rut of using the same equipment the same way for every workout, an occasional deviation can be just the way to jump-start your fitness.

The Least You Need to Know

➤ With 45 minutes, you can do some serious calorie burning.

➤ Use intervals sparingly to avoid overtraining.

➤ You can run, ride, or row your way to fitness.

➤ The elliptical trainer and cross-country ski machine are fine, no-impact alternatives to the usual run or ride.

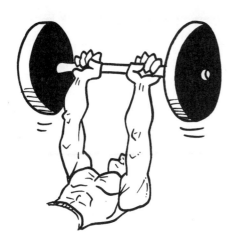

Chapter 15

The 45-Minute Strength-Training Workout

In This Chapter

➤ Forty-five minutes—enough for everything

➤ More mass for the upper body

➤ Squats—the do-everything leg exercise

➤ Pushing and pulling—using split routines

Now that we've graduated to 45 minutes of strength training, the compromises are gone. Three quarters of an hour is ample time to lift for even a dedicated athlete. In this chapter, we'll outline a few 45-minute routines that you can try depending on your goals. Whether your goal is to pump up your legs or your upper body or both, we've got a program for you. We also introduce you to split routines, a good way to squeeze even more muscle-building exercises into your busy schedule.

Upper-Body Emphasis

This first routine places extra emphasis on your upper body, but also introduces some new leg and midsection exercises that didn't make the cut in the 30-minute regimen. The inclusion of flyes and lateral raises in the mix adds some single-joint movements designed to isolate specific muscles. (Something that we didn't have the luxury of doing in just 30 minutes.) Once again, aim for sets of 10 to 12 reps (more if necessary for the midsection exercises) and limit your recovery between sets to two minutes.

Body Part	Exercise
Legs/hips	Leg press
	Leg extension
	Leg curl
Back	Lat pull down
	Upright rows
Chest	Chest press
	Flyes
Shoulders	Shoulder press
	Lateral raise
Arms	Seated biceps curl
	Triceps push down
Midsection	Reverse crunch
	Crunch
	Oblique crunch
	Back raise

Here is a rundown on each of the new exercises.

Flyes

Flyes are a great way to isolate the pecs. We'll instruct you on the free-weight version, but the pec deck machine, which duplicates the movement, is fine with us, too.

Lie on your back on a bench. Keep your feet flat on the floor or bend your knees and place your feet on the bench.

1. Start with a dumbbell in each hand, arms outstretched to the side.
2. Keep a slight bend in your elbows.
3. Slowly bring your arms together until the dumbbells lightly touch.
4. Squeeze at the top and then slowly return your arms to the starting position.

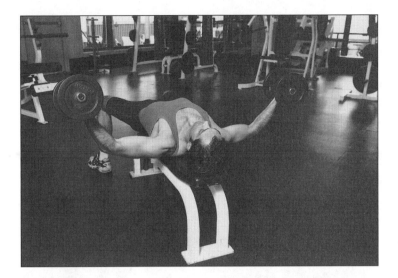

In the start/finish position, the elbows are slightly bent and the arms are outstretched.

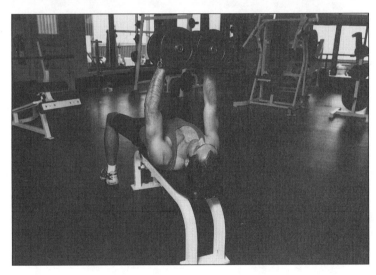

Contract your pecs and squeeze the dumbbells together at the top of the flye.

Flye Tips

Focus on form rather than using a lot of weight. Doing too much too soon (which always means too much weight) is a surefire way to injure yourself.

Don't lock your elbows.

Think of hugging a tree as you raise the weight through the range of motion.

Lateral Raises

Ever wonder why people wear shoulder pads in their clothes? Broadening your shoulders makes your waist look narrower. The lateral raise is a great exercise for isolating the deltoids (shoulders). Think of lateral raises as permanent shoulder pads. Here's what you need to know:

1. Stand with your feet shoulder width apart and your knees slightly bent.

2. Hold a dumbbell in each hand at your side with your palms facing in.

3. Keeping a slight bend in your elbow, and raise the dumbbells away from your sides until the arms are parallel to the floor.

4. Slowly return to the starting position.

In the start/finish position of the lateral raise, your arms are by your sides.

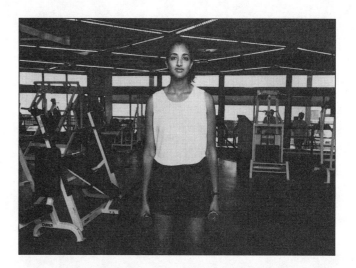

Keeping just a slight bend in your elbows, raise the dumbbells until your arms are parallel to the floor.

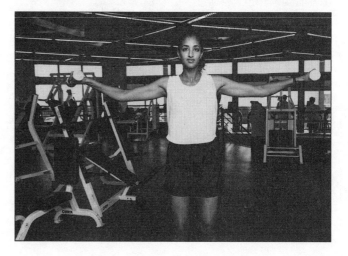

Oblique Crunch

As the name implies, the oblique crunch works the oblique muscles that surround your abdominals. They're involved in twisting movements and help stabilize your midsection. While there are several fancier and more impressive-looking exercises for your obliques, we consider this one the safest and most effective. Here's the proper form:

1. Lie on a mat with your left leg bent and your foot flat on the floor.

2. Place your right ankle so that it rests on top of your left knee.

3. Position your left hand behind your neck and keep your right hand outstretched.

4. Slowly curl up and twist toward your right knee.

5. Pause at the top and slowly return to the starting position.

6. Switch legs and arms and repeat on the other side.

Short Cuts

Remember that more is not better, and doing 10,000 reps of the oblique crunch will not burn off your love handles. That's where your cardio work and a good diet come in.

...our ab-
...es tight
...k pressed
...r in the
...n position.

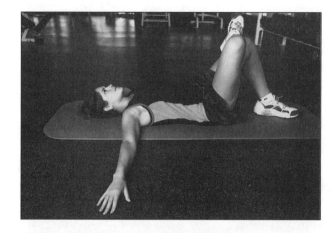

As you perform the oblique crunch, squeeze your shoulder towards the opposite knee.

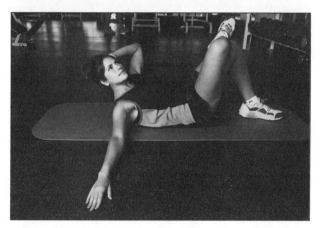

Lower-Body Emphasis

For those of you who want to give your legs an extra push, here's a routine for you. There are still lots for your upper body, but you can plan on your legs feeling this one as well. Remember, 10 to 12 reps per set and two minutes recovery between sets.

Body Part	Exercise
Legs/hips	Squat
	Leg extension
	Leg curl
	Abduction
	Adduction
	Standing calf raise
Back	Lat pull down

Body Part	Exercise
Chest	Chest press
Shoulders	Shoulder press
Arms	Seated biceps curl
	Triceps push down
Midsection	Reverse crunch
	Crunch
	Oblique crunch
	Back raise

We won't be heartbroken if you use the leg press instead of the squat—after all, it's a great exercise. When it comes to choosing one exercise that can help you make huge strength gains it's the squat. The downside is that you can overdo it and mess up a variety of body parts.

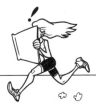

Info to Go

Squats are widely considered to be the single best, most effective exercise you can do for your legs. While we love them, it's especially important that you pay close attention to your form as you squat. One of the most common mistakes we see in the weight room is lifters piling on much too much weight and only doing a "quarter squat." We prefer that you go down until your thighs are parallel to the floor. This greater range of motion does a better job of strengthening the muscles, yet allows you to use less weight in the process.

Squat

The squat is a very challenging exercise that demands strict attention to form. Though we've said it throughout the book with other exercises (and we definitely mean it), form here is essential. Here's what you need to know:

1. Stand underneath the barbell with your feet slightly wider than shoulder width apart.

2. With your arms holding the barbell with a grip about six to eight inches from your shoulders, lift the barbell off the rack.

3. Take one step backward so you don't hit the racks as you squat. Keep your toes pointed slightly outward.

4. Keeping your back straight, begin to bend your knees until your thighs are parallel to the floor. Don't squat deeper. However, if you squat too little, you're not maximizing the benefits of the exercise. A greater range of motion ensures full strength gains.

5. Return to your starting position.

Squat Tips

Keep your weight on your heels, not your toes.

Maintain an upright posture.

Keep your abdominals tight.

Always inhale deeply as you descend; exhale as you ascend.

Place the bar across your upper back, not on your neck.

Always squat with a spotter or safety rack.

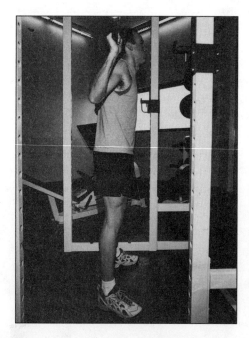

Note the flat back and upright posture in the start/finish position.

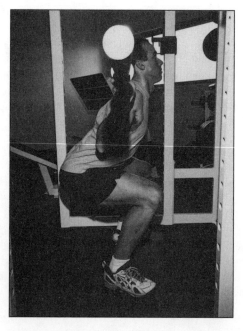

At the bottom position of the squat, the thighs are parallel to the ground and the knees stay behind the toes.

Abduction

Your hip abductor muscles are the muscles of your outer thigh that move your leg sideways. We'll show you the exercise using a machine, but the calisthenics version (possibly with an ankle weight) is fine too. (Women should keep in mind that when you work a muscle, it grows, so don't do hip abduction if you think they are going to make your thighs slimmer.)

1. Sit on the machine with your back against the back pad and your outer legs against the thigh pads.
2. Secure the belt if there is one.
3. Push the legs apart as far as possible by pushing against the thigh pads.
4. Return slowly to the initial starting position.

Abduction Tips

Keep an erect posture during the exercise.

Maintain control of the weight stack at all times; don't allow it to slam as you return to the starting position.

Keep your abdominals tight.

Keep your head and trunk against the back pad.

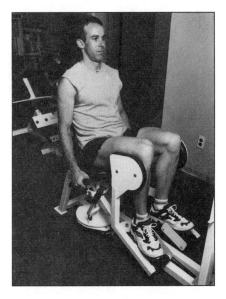

Abduction begins and ends with your legs together.

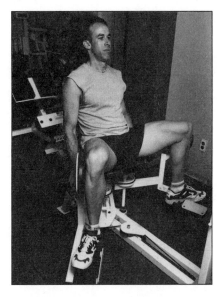

Using the muscles of your outer thigh, bring your legs out as far as possible.

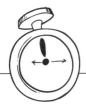

Short Cuts

While we find machines much more effective for abduction and adduction, you can do the floor exercises so common to aerobics classes at home.

Adduction

The adductors do the opposite of the abductors: bring your legs inward. Since they're small muscles, there's no need to do tons of work for them. Nevertheless they come in handy for those of you who are active in sports that require lateral movement such as tennis or basketball. If no machine is available, the exercise mat awaits you. On the machine, here's the scoop:

1. Sit on the machine with your back against the back pad and your inner legs against the thigh pads.
2. Secure the belt if there is one.
3. Bring the legs together as close as possible by pushing against the thigh pads.
4. Return slowly to the initial starting position.

Adduction Tips

Keep your abdominals tight.

Keep your head and trunk against the back pad.

Maintain control of the weight stack.

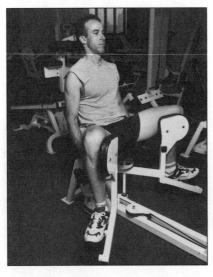

Adduction exercises begin and end with the legs apart.

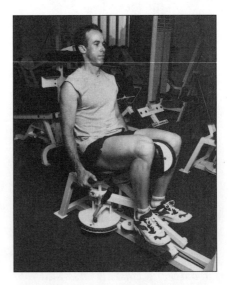

Check the position of your legs.

Standing Calf Raise

If you want to walk up stairs with a little pep in your step, you'd better begin to strengthen those gastrocnemius muscles of your calves that help spring you up on to your toes.

1. Stand on the bottom step so that the balls of your feet are on the edge of the step and the heels extend over the edge.

2. Position your shoulders beneath the pads, and place your hands on either side of the pads.

3. Keeping your legs straight, rise up onto the toes as high as possible.

4. Return slowly to a position where your heels are hanging down as far as possible. This will provide a good stretch.

Standing Calf Raise Tips

Keep your back straight, don't arch it.

Maintain a steady up and down motion—no rocking back and forth.

Perform each repetition slowly.

Keep your abdominals tight.

Keep your legs straight.

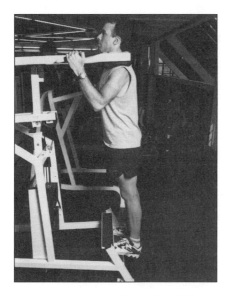

In order to exercise through a full range of motion, start the exercise with your heels below your toes.

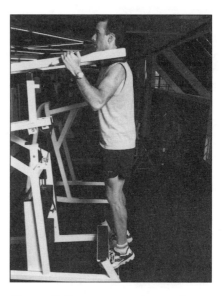

Come all the way up onto your toes at the top of the motion.

177

Split Personality

As we've told you, we generally prefer full-body routines; however, *split routines* are a sound alternative—especially if you want to get in extra exercises for each body part.

Here are a couple of split scenarios that should be effective and challenging. The most common configuration for a split routine—and the one we like best—is the push/pull split. This routine splits your upper body into "pulling" and "pushing" muscles. The pulling muscles include the muscles of your back (lats, trapeius, rhomboids) and biceps. Working these muscles on the same day is key since your biceps assist in most exercises for your back (pull downs and rows, for example). Similarly, the pushing muscles of the chest (pecs), shoulders (delts), and triceps are grouped together.

In our less-than-humble opinion, split routines that work the pecs and triceps on consecutive days, or back and biceps (scenarios we've seen quite often), don't make sense. Whether you like it or not, your triceps are involved in all pressing movements such as the bench press, incline press, shoulder press, and so on. So, for example, if Monday is your "chest day," your triceps will still be recovering on Tuesday. Working them again in your next split session will be counterproductive. Worse yet, if you work out your arms on Monday and try to do a workout for your chest on Tuesday, your triceps will be so sapped that they'll be unable to do the necessary work for your pressing movements.

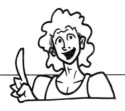

Workout Words

A **split routine** is a training plan in which you divide your workout over two or more days. Split routines are especially effective if you want to do more than a few exercises per body part.

It might sound complicated at first, and it is a tad bit more confusing than a Monday, Wednesday, Friday workout regimen in which you do the same workout each day; however, once you get the hang of it it's no more complicated than following a recipe.

Dividing your body up as described above gives a configuration like this:

➤ Days one and four: chest, shoulders, triceps, midsection.

➤ Days two and five: legs, back, biceps.

Days One and Four

Let's get started!

Body Part	Exercise
Chest	Chest press
	Incline press

Body Part	Exercise
Chest	Decline press
	Flyes
Shoulders	Military press
	Lateral raises
Triceps	Triceps push down
	Triceps kickback
Midsection	Crunch
	Oblique crunch
	Reverse crunch
	Back raise

Since we're only doing half your body, there's room to introduce some more new exercises.

Incline Press

The incline press works on the upper part of your pecs and is a good complement to the bench press.

1. Lie down on the incline bench and place your feet either flat on the floor or on the footrest (if one is present).
2. Grab the bar with a grip slightly wider apart than shoulder width.
3. Lift the bar from the uprights or have a spotter assist you.
4. Slowly lower until it touches the upper part of your chest, just below your collar bone; then slowly return to the initial starting position.

Incline Press Tips

Make sure you don't lock out your elbows as you straighten your arms.

Keep your back flat against the bench.

Keep your head on the bench.

Keep your buttocks on the bench.

Lower the bar gently to your chest; don't bounce the bar off of your chest.

Keep your feet and legs still.

Keep your abdominals tight.

Don't hold your breath.

179

In the start/finish position, your elbows should be slightly bent.

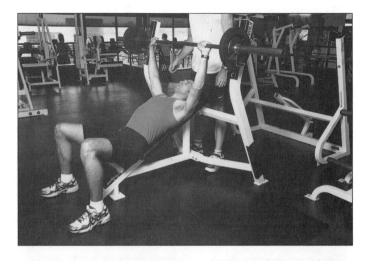

Slowly, bring the bar down to just below your collarbone.

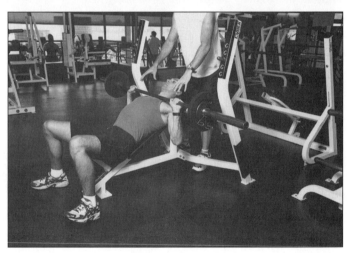

Decline Press

The decline bench works the lower part of your chest. Essentially you follow the same procedure as the flat and incline bench.

1. Lie down on the bench, putting your feet under the support provided.
2. Grab the bar with a grip slightly wider apart than shoulder width.
3. Lift from the upright or have a spotter assist you.
4. Slowly lower the bar to your chest just below the nipple line; then return to the initial starting position.

Decline Press Tips

Make sure you don't lock out your elbows as you straighten your arms.

Keep your back flat against the bench.

Keep your head on the bench.

Lower the bar gently to your chest; don't bounce the bar off of your chest.

Keep your abdominals tight.

Don't hold your breath.

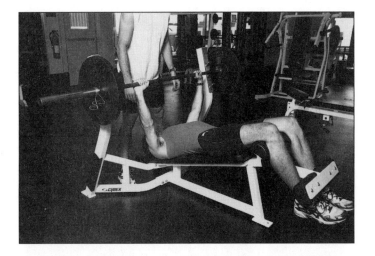

For the decline press, you begin and end with your arms extended.

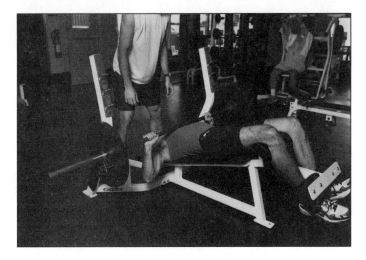

Once again, the bar should be lowered to your chest in a slow, controlled fashion.

Triceps Kickback

The triceps kickback is a great way to isolate your triceps, but it requires strict form to be effective. All too often we see people throwing around much more weight than they can handle and using horrible form in the process.

1. Place one knee and hand on the bench for support.

2. Slightly bend the standing leg.

3. The working arm should be bent to 90° at the shoulder and 90° at the elbow.

4. Keep your arm close to your side. To gain the full benefit from this exercise, it's important to keep your upper arm parallel to the ground. Pay strict attention to your form.

5. Slowly straighten your elbow and return to the starting position.

Triceps Kickback Tips

Make sure your back doesn't sag.

Make sure you don't shift your body back and forth in an effort to get the weight up.

Don't allow the upper arm to drop—keep it parallel to the ground throughout the range of motion.

Keep your back straight and your abdominals tight.

Keep your eyes fixed on the bench. Looking up or sideways can put stress on your neck.

Begin the triceps kickback with your arm at a right angle.

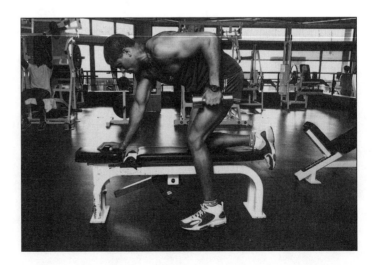

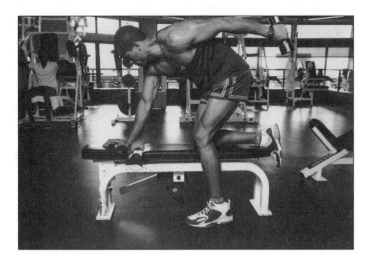

Straighten your elbow without letting your upper arm drop.

Days Two and Five

Days two and five are dedicated to legs, back, and biceps. Make sure you separate these exercises by a couple of days to avoid overtraining.

Body Part	Exercise
Legs/hips	Leg press
	Leg extension
	Leg curl
	Abduction
	Adduction
	Standing calf raise
Back	Lat pull down
	Dumbbell row
	Upright row
	Shrug
Biceps	Seated biceps curl
	Concentration curl

Once again, we've introduced a couple more new exercises.

Dumbbell Rows

Dumbbell rows emphasize the lats, middle traps, and rhomboids. They're great exercises to help broaden your back.

183

1. Place the left hand and the left knee on a bench and position the right foot on the floor at a comfortable distance from the bench.
2. Reach down with the right hand and grab the dumbbell.
3. Lift the dumbbell off the floor, keeping the right arm straight. The right palm should be facing the bench.
4. Keeping the upper arm near the torso, slowly pull the dumbbell up to the right shoulder as if you were sawing a piece of wood.
5. Pause briefly and gradually return the dumbbell to the starting position.
6. Repeat with the left arm (with the right hand and right knee on the bench).

Dumbbell Row Tips

Maintain a straight back; don't arch it.

Don't allow your shoulder to move excessively.

Don't swing your body in an effort to get the weight up.

Don't allow your torso to twist.

Keep your abdominals tight.

Keep your shoulder and torso down and parallel to the floor.

Begin the exercise with your arm straight and your torso facing the ground.

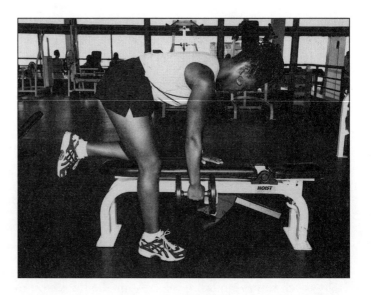

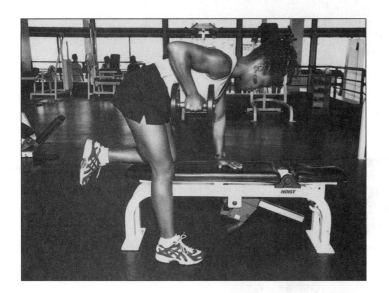

Pull your elbow up high, without twisting your torso.

Shrugs

Shrugs are the best way to isolate the traps, the muscle that surrounds your neck. For anyone involved in contact sports or activities where neck and head injuries are a possibility, the added neck stability that shrugs can develop can be crucial.

1. Stand with your feet shoulder width apart.
2. Hold the barbell wider apart than shoulder width with palms facing your thighs.
3. Keeping your arms and legs straight, move the bar as high as possible by trying to touch your shoulders to your ears.
4. Pause briefly and slowly return to the initial starting position.

Shrug Tips

Don't allow the range of motion to decrease as you get tired.

Don't rock your body back and forth in an effort to lift the weight.

Keep your abdominals tight and your back erect without leaning backward.

You can perform this exercise with either a barbell or a dumbbell for a change of pace.

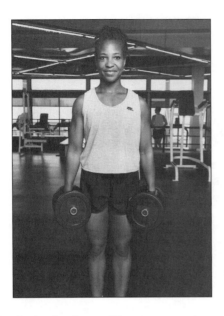
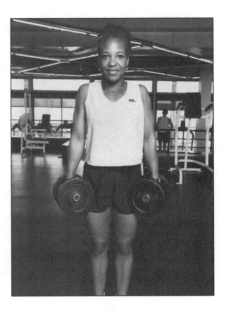

Begin the shrug with your arms at your sides and your shoulders down.

As you perform the exercise, pull your shoulders up as high as possible.

Concentration Curls

Concentration curls are a great way to ensure that you use strict form on your curls. Since they are a little harder, you can expect to use less weight than you are accustomed to on other biceps exercises.

1. With a dumbbell in your hand, sit on a bench and lean forward and rest your arm on the inner part of your thigh.
2. Your palm should be facing your opposite thigh.
3. Raise the dumbbell by slowly bending to a point just short of your shoulder.
4. Lower the dumbbell slowly, straightening your elbow to the starting position.

Concentration Curls Tips

Don't lean or rock backward and forward in an effort to hoist the dumbbell up—you could hurt your back. If your form isn't perfect, immediately lessen the weight.

Make sure you don't move your leg from side to side in an effort to help you lift the weight.

Keep your abdominals tight and your back erect as you are leaning forward.

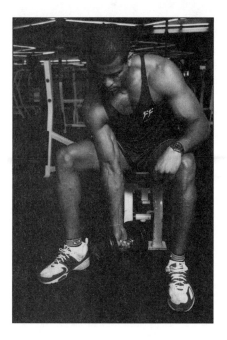

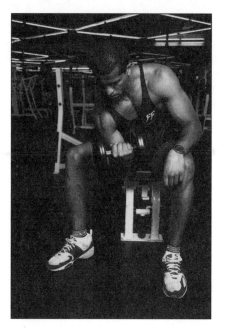

Make sure your elbow is braced against your thigh.

Curl the weight up without leaning back.

The Least You Need to Know

➤ Forty-five minutes is more than enough time to do a comprehensive upper-body and lower-body routine.

➤ Moving from 30 to 45 minutes, there are more exercises in your bag of tricks to keep you from getting bored.

➤ Squats are a great overall-strengthening exercise.

➤ Split routines let you expand your training program.

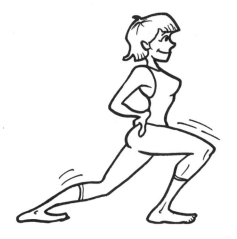

The 60-Minute Workout

In Chapter 13, "The 45-Minute Workout," we outlined a 45-minute routine that includes stretching, cardio, and strength training, sandwiched by a warm-up and cooldown. While we're confident that a 45-minute workout is sufficient, a little more time would come in handy. The additional 15 minutes allows for an extra five sets of strength-training exercises and another 10 minutes or so of cardio work.

As the fitness coordinator for the New York City Police Department, Jonathan has had an army of cops come to him and say, "I've got 60 minutes to work out each day during my lunch hour. What should I do in that limited amount of time?" Jonathan usually gives a slow and knowing nod, asks if they want to cover the "Big Three" (strength, cardio, and stretching), and spits out an exercise routine to help them get or stay in shape. Don't let this talk of cops fool you—before you get the image of Andy Sipowitz wolfing down a doughnut and coffee, you should know that most of the models pictured in this book come from Jonathan's gym.

It's About Time

Here's a thumbnail sketch of how to break down your 60-minute workout. There's room to tweak these figures depending on what you want to improve most—feel free to bump up the cardio to 30 minutes and cut a few strength-training exercises (try the routine we used in Chapter 13) or add a few extra sets of muscle building and sacrifice five minutes of running or riding.

➤ Warm-up (5 minutes).

➤ Cardiovascular (20 minutes).

➤ Cooldown (5 minutes).

➤ Strength training (25 minutes).

➤ Stretch (5 minutes).

Our chief aim in this chapter is to show you how economical and effective you can be in a still relatively modest amount of time. Once you come to see that you can address your major fitness needs without taking out a time-share at Muscle Beach, you're more likely to stick with a regimen that makes a difference.

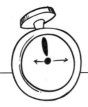

Short Cuts

For those of you with limited gym time, there's one more great thing about the VersaClimber—it's one of the most underused pieces of equipment in the gym. While this may not please the VersaClimber sales staff, it can be to your advantage. The next time you're at the gym during peak time, impatiently tapping your feet, rolling your eyes, and staring at your watch while waiting for a treadmill to become available, give the VersaClimber a try instead.

The Workout

In the expanded 60-minute workout, the basic structure of your workout remains the same; only the timing varies. As before, remember to warm up for five minutes or so to get some blood pumping and your joints lubricated. A light sweat is all you're looking for.

Once you're warmed up, you can move on to your cardio work. As we've stressed before, the key to getting the most out of your cardiovascular workout is exercising at the correct intensity, so get those heart-rate monitors ready and make sure your heart's pumping at at least 70 percent of its max. Any of the exercise modes that we've already discussed—walking, jogging, cycling, rowing—will do just fine, but the list of great equipment doesn't end there.

Going Up?

If you want a change of pace, try out the elliptical trainer or cross-country ski machine or challenge yourself with the VersaClimber, a full-body climbing exercise guaranteed to remove any lingering doubts you might have about whether 20 minutes of cardiovascular sweating is really enough.

Working out on the VersaClimber feels like climbing an endless ladder and puts both your upper and lower body musculature to work to provide a tremendous cardiovascular workout. A few years back, when Jonathan got a big idea in his little head about setting some ridiculous 24-hour stair-climbing record, he did workouts of up to two hours on the VersaClimber. (He assures us that it seemed like a good idea at the time.) Unless you share Jonathan's *Guinness Book of World Records* aspirations, a far more modest time frame will suit you just fine.

The VersaClimber is an intimidating piece of equipment even to many regulars (perhaps in part due to its resemblance to a medieval torture device). In truth, while it can be a killer workout, it doesn't always have to be. Remember that, unlike a treadmill that will spit you off the back if you don't keep up, the VersaClimber only moves as fast as you make it go, so there's no one but you to blame if the workout is too hard. Another nice feature of the VersaClimber is that by using both your arms and your legs, you'll find it easy to elevate your heart rate to within your training zone without too much stress on any individual muscles.

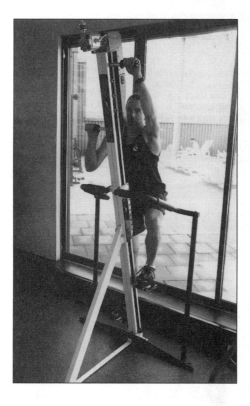

The VersaClimber gives a great cardiovascular workout.

Sitting Down on the Job

While the VersaClimber is one of the most intimidating pieces of equipment in the gym, the recumbent bike is firmly planted at the opposite end of the spectrum. Most

191

people look at the recumbent and figure that any exercise that takes place in the same position that you're in to watch a football game can only be so challenging. And while it's true that some exercisers expend more energy opening their designer bottled water in the middle of their workout than they do on the recumbent, it can be a legitimate training tool, especially for people with back pain that prevents them from riding a conventional bike. In other words, like most anything else, you'll get out what you put in.

If you've resisted spending a lot of time working out on a conventional upright bike, either because of back pain or because you find the discomfort of a standard bicycle seat more trouble than it's worth, we suggest giving a recumbent a try. The muscles that you use to pedal (mostly your quads, glutes, and hamstrings, along with some help from your calf muscles) are the same regardless of whether you're on an upright or recumbent bike, and assuming that you elevate your heart rate to the same level, your caloric expenditure and cardiovascular benefit will be comparable as well. In other words, remember that it's a piece of exercise equipment, not a La-Z-Boy recliner, and the recumbent can provide a challenging workout.

Once again, since your cardio time is limited, the key is to get the most out of your workouts. Most machines in the gym, including the StairMaster, Life-cycle, elliptical trainers and most treadmills have programs built into their fancy, high-tech electronic monitors. As we've mentioned, many of these programs have fancy names like "cardio blaster," but they're usually nothing more than loosely disguised interval training workouts that automatically vary the intensity of your workouts.

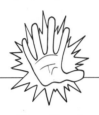

Stop Short

Finally, don't forget to cool down for a few minutes after your cardio workout. Check your pulse one more time to make sure your heart rate is down below 100 or so.

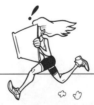

Info to Go

While most people think of them in the gym, recumbent road bikes have been around for decades and have a cultlike following among some riders. In fact, they've even been ridden up Mt. Washington, New Hampshire, a 7.6-mile climb with an average grade of over 12 percent.

In Chapter 13 we alluded to a few of our favorite programs including the LifeCycle Hill Profile and the StairMaster Lunar Landing. Either of them can be used within your 60-minute workout, as can some of the other programs on these machines. For those of you with a short attention span, the LifeCycle also has a "Random" program that varies the intensity every 10 seconds for as long as you pedal. The StairMaster also has several other programs such as the "Roller Coaster" and "Pikes Peak," either of which we like.

Lifting

Having moved from 45 to 60 minutes, we've added 10 minutes to the lifting segment of your workout, which translates to an extra five exercises, based on one minute per exercise with a one-minute recovery. This allows for the inclusion of a little more ab work as well as exercises specifically for your biceps and triceps. Even with the extra exercises, it's a fairly short program, so the key to your success is intensity. Don't just stop at 10 or 12 as if it's a magic number—do as many as you can without sacrificing form or safety. When you can do more than 12 reps, it's time to increase the weight by about 5 percent. Walk your way through a few easy sets and you might as well just skip it.

Here is a pair of 13 set routines you can do—one with an extra emphasis on your upper body, and one stressing your legs. Regardless of which routine you choose, as before, you'll move from larger to smaller muscles, performing sets of 10 to 12 reps. Remember to concentrate on slow, controlled reps (three seconds positive, three seconds negative with a pause in between).

Leg Emphasis

- ❏ Leg press.
- ❏ Leg extension.
- ❏ Leg curl.
- ❏ Standing calf raise.
- ❏ Seated calf raise.
- ❏ Chest press.
- ❏ Lat pull down.
- ❏ Shoulder press.
- ❏ Biceps curl.
- ❏ Triceps extension.
- ❏ Reverse crunch.
- ❏ Crunch.
- ❏ Oblique crunch.

Upper-Body Emphasis

- ❏ Leg press.
- ❏ Standing calf raise.
- ❏ Chest press.
- ❏ Row.
- ❏ Dip (or assisted dip on Gravitron)
- ❏ Upright row.
- ❏ Lat pull down.
- ❏ Triceps extension.
- ❏ Biceps curl.
- ❏ Reverse crunch.
- ❏ Crunch.
- ❏ Oblique crunch.
- ❏ Shoulder press.

The inclusion of "only" three ab exercises is also noteworthy. Quite often, trainers advocate far more exercises and many gyms even offer "ab classes" that run as long as 20 or even 30 minutes. While we fully understand and appreciate the need for strong abdominal muscles—lower back injury prevention, improved sports performance, and appearance are among the most prominent—there's no need to go overboard and spend too much of your valuable time doing ab work. Also keep in mind that there's no such thing as *spot reduction,* so all the crunches in the world won't burn the fat around your midsection. Unless you're down to your "fighting weight," your "six-pack" will be obscured by a layer of fat.

Stretching the Truth

Forgive us for sounding like a broken record, but some things bear repeating. Jonathan, the exercise physiologist of our team, has heard all the excuses you could imagine for not stretching ("I'll do it when I get home," "I'm naturally limber," and, "Stretching is for sissies" are his favorites). Deidre, our resident physical therapist, has treated patients for a variety of ailments caused by poor flexibility (lower back pain, Iliotibial Band Syndrome, and hamstring pulls are among the most common). While this may be bad for Deidre's practice, we urge you to stretch after every workout. As we told you in Chapter 7, "Start with Stretching," make sure to hold your stretches for 20 to 30 seconds, don't bounce when you stretch, and never stretch to the point of pain. The same five stretches that we suggested in Chapter 13 (groin stretch, hip stretch, seated hamstring stretch, quadriceps stretch, and standing calf stretch) will do just fine here. If you have a few extra minutes, feel free to throw in a few more stretches. We'd recommend the lunge and lower back/hip stretches described in Chapter 7.

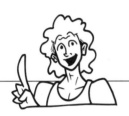

Workout Words

Spot reduction is a disproved theory that refers to burning fat specifically around the exercising muscle. In fact, the muscles that are used during an exercise have no effect on the pattern of fat loss.

By now, a full 60 minutes to exercise may seem like a luxury. With that hour you can effectively and efficiently address all your major fitness needs. Be sure to adhere to the principles we've outlined and you're guaranteed to see significant improvements in your strength, flexibility, and cardiovascular fitness.

The Least You Need to Know

➤ An hour is plenty of time for a full workout.

➤ Using the VersaClimber or recumbent bike can bring some variety to your routine.

➤ Like it or not, you can't skip the warm-up, cooldown, or stretching.

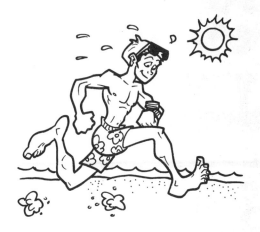

Chapter 17

The 60-Minute Cardio Workout

> ### In This Chapter
>
> ➤ One-hour workouts can train you to run a marathon
>
> ➤ The short workout marathon program
>
> ➤ Riding your way to a new century
>
> ➤ Classes can help an hour speed by

In the previous 16 chapters, we've given you scores of tips on how to get the best workout in the shortest amount of time. Now that we've graduated to a 60-minute cardio workout, we have ample time to turn you into an even fitter fat-burning machine able to leap tall buildings in a single bound. (Well, at least we'll get you to the top of the building taking two steps at a time.)

In past chapters, we've made tongue-in-cheek references to the things that you can't do with short workouts—you can't earn a berth on the Olympics team and you'll have to put your professional bodybuilding career on hold. Now, instead of telling you what you can't do, let's focus on what *is* possible with 60-minute cardiovascular workouts. The answer is, lots.

Want to run a marathon? Want to ride a century (100 miles) on your bike? We can do that. Even if you'd rather eat moldy bread than run 26.2 miles in one chunk, logging hour-long cardio workouts will have you looking and feeling great. In fact, no matter how ambitious your goals, you can get there with a training regimen built around one-hour workouts.

In this chapter we'll discuss some of the many ways you can use your hour to meet a variety of fitness goals.

Run for Your Life

Many of you may have raised your eyebrows when we suggested that you could run a marathon based around 60 minutes a day of training. That's natural. After all, most people take three to five hours to run a marathon and world-class runners take over two hours to cover the distance. No, we're not suggesting that you'll be going to run stride for stride with the top Kenyans at the next Boston Marathon. (In fact, on 25 hours of training per week you're not likely to run with those fleet-footed guys.) Nor do we want you to think that you won't ever have to run more than 60 minutes at a time to complete a marathon with a degree of grace. However, we are telling you that you can successfully complete a marathon with far less training and far fewer long runs than you might expect.

Every November, your coauthors stroll from their Brooklyn homes to watch the New York City Marathon. (At least during the years that none of us are running it.) After the 1998 race, one of Jonathan's coworkers, who had never run before, was so inspired by the grand human procession that she decided that she wanted to give it a go. While resolving to run the marathon the day after the race is as common as swearing off booze on the morning on January 1, this woman was so passionate that Jonathan offered to help her prepare. Twelve months later, having followed a very reasonable training program that never exceeded seven hours a week of running, Jonathan stood under the finish line gloating like a proud parent as she ran across the finish in Central Park. Her time was over four hours, about two hours behind the female winner, Adriana Fernandez, but she'd run the whole way and had a memorable experience.

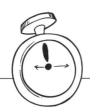

Short Cuts

Obviously, if you don't run on a regular basis the thought of running 26 miles, 385 yards is an exercise in masochism. So by all means, please start with more moderate goals. A logical progression is to fix your sights on completing a few 5K (3.1-mile) races. Next, try a few 5-milers and/or 10Ks (6.2 miles). Next, if you're feeling up to it, try a half marathon (13.1 miles).

Training for a Marathon

However, as we just mentioned, if your goal is to get to the marathon starting line healthy and to finish the race that way, the minimal amount of training that's required to finish is far more modest than what you might think.

First, you'll need to *gradually* work your way up to a total of 20 miles per week. If you've been running less than that, avoid the temptation to immediately jump up to 20 miles. That's a quick recipe for overuse injuries. A good guideline to keep in mind is that you should never increase your weekly mileage by more than 10 percent. That means that if you've been running three or four miles a day every other day, you should increase your weekly mileage by only one mile per week until you reach 20. Again, increasing your mileage more drastically is too much too soon, so while we're glad you're eager to do more, harness your enthusiasm and increase you mileage slowly. (By the way, that reminds us of the simple fact that you can't finish the race if you can't make it to the starting line.)

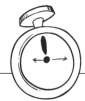

Short Cuts

Runners often struggle with the dilemma of whether to run when they're sick. While missing workouts can be frustrating, it's preferable to making yourself even sicker. While your doctor should have the final say, we like the "neck" rule. If your symptoms are above your neck—congestion, runny nose, headache—an easy run probably won't hurt and may even make you feel better. If your ailments include chest congestion, sore throat, or other symptoms below your head, hit the couch, hammer the vitamin C, and read a good book. (If you're really having "runner's withdrawal," read in your running shoes.)

Once you work up to 20 miles per week, maintain that distance until about four months from the day of the marathon. According to the New York Road Runners Club, the organizers of this huge running parade (now the biggest marathon in the world), "Novice and casual marathoners should gradually build to a peak of 30 to 40 miles per week, which they hold for at least six to eight weeks."

If you've managed to do that—and stay healthy—here's a training plan for the last four months leading up to race day. Jonathan has used this program with several first timers (including Deidre) and each one of them crossed the line injury free, without walking. As you'll see, there are only a handful of workouts of over an hour.

The most important factors in this schedule are the total weekly mileage and the "long run." Do your best to match figures and don't worry too much if you have to juggle some of the other days around.

Here's a weird thing to say in a chapter that's discussing the virtues of running a marathon. In our opinion, too many runners feel a need to run a marathon as if it's some rite of passage that every runner has to go through to really be part of "the club." If you don't have an urge to put yourself through the rigors of training and racing, then we see no reason for you to do what it takes to run 26 continuous miles. On the other hand, if you often find yourself wondering, "Can I cover the distance?" we hope we're able to convince you that while the long training runs can be arduous, running a marathon doesn't mean that you have to mortgage the farm to complete the distance.

Training Program for a Marathon

Weeks to Go	Saturday	Sunday	Monday	Tuesday	Wednesday	Thursday	Friday	Weekly Total Miles
17	3	6	0	4	4	0	3	20
16	3	7	0	4	4	0	4	22
15	3	8	0	4	5	0	4	24
14	3	9	0	3	3	0	3	21
13	4	10	0	4	3	0	3	24
12	4	11	0	5	3	0	3	26
11	4	12	0	5	4	0	3	28
10	0	14	0	3	0	0	3	20
9	4	16	0	3	0	0	3	26
8	4	12	0	5	4	0	3	28
7	4	18	0	3	3	0	3	31
6	3	14	0	3	0	0	3	23
5	3	20	0	3	3	0	3	32
4	4	16	0	5	5	0	5	35
3	6	20	0	4	4	0	4	38
2	6	14	0	3	0	0	3	26
1	6	0	5	0	4	0	3	18
0	Walk	Race						

Marathon Training Tips

Reduce your mileage or take a day off if you are injured or ill.

Stretch regularly. Tight muscles are the biggest cause of shin splints and other overuse injuries.

If you miss a workout due to illness or injury, don't try to make it up. Chalk it up to the gods of rest and do your next schedule workout. Many conscientious people who miss workouts try and double up the next day. Nice idea, but it generally means you'll be too tired the following day and that leads to all sorts of maladies such as injury and burnout.

Don't worry about the pace that other people are running—avoid the temptation o speed up if a "rabbit" goes by you in training. He or she might be out for half the distance that you're covering or simply be faster.

Stretch. Oh yeah, we said it before, but it's worth repeating.

Make sure you wear good running shoes. Remember to replace them approximately every 500 miles.

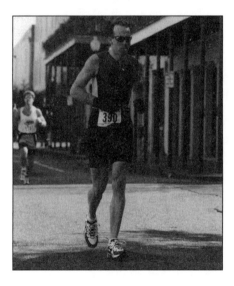

Jonathan doing his best to hide his joy at the Mardi Gras Marathon in New Orleans.

Check with your local running club or try www.coolrunning.com for a comprehensive list of marathons throughout the country.

Time for a Ride

While becoming a competitive cyclist is a time-consuming endeavor, an hour bike ride is ample time to do some serious riding. For many racing cyclists, completing the standard 40-kilometer (24.8-mile) time trial distance (a time trial is a solo race against the clock) in under an hour is a major accomplishment. For other riders, simply keeping your cranks turning for 60 minutes is an accomplishment.

Training for a Century Ride

Another major milestone for cyclists is riding a century—100 miles—in one day. (A metric century, though not quite as ambitious, is still a standard benchmark ride. That's 62 miles to you nonmetric fans.) While each event requires a fair amount of training (and a forgiving bike saddle), neither one is out of reach even if you're short on time. As with the marathon program we just outlined, you can give it an honest effort doing mostly 60-minute workouts, though you'll need some long-distance training rides to round out your training. Again, if riding a century gets you as excited as drinking stale coffee, don't worry. We're just trying to show you that an hour on a bike is plenty of time even if you do have ambitious goals.

Here's a sample training program for those of you preparing to ride your first century. One ride each week needs to be more than an hour long; as long as you can free up some extra time on the weekend, you should be fine.

In Chapter 24, "Seasonal Workouts," we'll tell you a little more about the different types of bikes that are available, but for long-distance rides such as a century, a road or touring bike is definitely your best bet. The fat tires of a mountain bike or even a hybrid are great for negotiating rough terrain, but unless you're got the stamina of Samson, it's not an efficient way to go if you want to ride a century in less than a century.

Century Ride Tips

Get yourself a pair of good padded cycling shorts. Expect to pay anywhere from $30 to $80 for a good pair.

Rarely will you have a closer relationship with an inanimate object than with your bicycle saddle. Experiment with a few different designs and don't try to save a few bucks by purchasing a bargain brand.

Always keep your tires inflated to their rated pressure. Underinflated tires are more prone to flats and are slower than tires that are properly inflated.

Familiarize yourself with the basics of bicycle mechanics. You should at least know how to repair a flat tire and adjust your gears and breaks.

Unless you're planning to race, don't worry if your bike weighs an extra pound or two. We're always amazed at riders who are 5 to 10 pounds overweight, but think nothing of spending an extra $500 for a lightweight pair of wheels.

Century rides are popular throughout the country. Check with *Bicycling* magazine or www.bicycling.com for a list of long-distance rides.

Training for a Century Ride

Weeks to Go	Saturday (Long Easy Ride)	Sunday	Monday	Tuesday (Intervals)	Wednesday	Thursday (Hills)	Friday
12	25 miles	1 hour	Rest	1 hour	Rest	1 hour	30 minutes
11	30 miles	1 hour	Rest	1 hour	Rest	1 hour	35 minutes
10	35 miles	1 hour	Rest	1 hour	Rest	1 hour	40 minutes
9	40 miles	1 hour	Rest	1 hour	Rest	1 hour	45 minutes
8	45 miles	1 hour	Rest	1 hour	30 minutes	1 hour	50 minutes
7	50 miles	1 hour	Rest	1 hour	35 minutes	1 hour	55 minutes
6	60 miles	1 hour	Rest	1 hour	40 minutes	1 hour	1 hour
5	60 miles	1 hour	Rest	1 hour	45 minutes	1 hour	1 hour
4	65 miles	1 hour	Rest	1 hour	50 minutes	1 hour	1 hour
3	70 miles	1 hour	Rest	1 hour	55 minutes	1 hour	1 hour
2	75 miles	1 hour	Rest	1 hour	1 hour	1 hour	1 hour
1	80 miles	1 hour	Rest	45 minutes	Rest	Easy spin	Rest
0	100 miles						

Show Some Class

In the good old days when Jane Fonda was diva of the fitness world, taking an exercise class meant throwing on a leotard, a pair of leg warmers, and going to an "aerobics" or aerobic dance class. Since then, classes evolved to include "body shaping" or "sculpting" classes. Next came step classes, spin classes, and more. Today there are more classes available than excuses not to take them. While we love the discipline of solo workouts, there's something to be said for working out in a group setting. Whether it's the music, the teacher, or the other poor slobs sweating up a storm around you—or all of the above—many people find a class to be very motivating and fun. Think of "misery loves company" and "one for all and all for one" and you've got the clichés to capture the power of group dynamics. Even Joe, a member of the U.S. marathon kayak team, who regularly trains alone, is amazed when he works out with other paddlers how much harder he pushes himself. It's not that he wasn't trying on his own—he was!—it's just human nature to squeeze out that extra effort when surrounded by others.

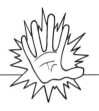

Stop Short

While we're big proponents of group classes, beware: Some classes we've seen in fitness centers are heavier on style than substance, better suited for Broadway dancers than those of us who can't handle anything trickier than walking and chewing gum simultaneously. Having said that, most of them that we've seen or done are worth checking out to see if you like them.

Another note: Exercise classes tend to run 50 to 55 minutes. Though we've included cardio classes in our 60-minute section, many shorter options are available as well.

Spin Your Wheels

As we've already told you, indoor group cycling, generically known as "spinning," has become very popular over the past few years in gyms across the country. While spinning was the original, several other companies now offer instructor certifications and specialized bikes for use in class settings. Even StairMaster has gotten into the act with its RevMaster bike—endorsed by three-time Tour de France winner Greg LeMond. Jonathan and several of his teammates take spinning classes during the off-season when the weather is too hostile, so you can be sure that these classes are well suited to athletes and recreational riders alike.

If you haven't taken one of these classes, you should, since they can get pretty wild, and considering how hard your heart is beating, quite fun. An hour of group cycling is both challenging and a great way to make the time fly by. For those of you who enjoy pumping music and the encouragement that a teacher and a group setting can provide, spinning is a great option. One word of caution: If you haven't done any cycling (indoors or out) in a while, don't jump into a class and hammer away. That's a good way to be massively stiff the next day; or worse, get injured.

Step to the Beat

Here's one you may not have heard of before: classes on a StairMaster. The classes, called "stomp," are a great way to add a little pep to your usual StairMaster workout. Again, one of the best features is that a well-led class will make the time go by faster. Stomp classes were introduced in New York City in summer 1999 and have gained popularity steadily since. As with any other type of class, the format varies slightly from teacher to teacher, but there are few basics that you can safely expect at any stomp class.

➤ Music with a strong beat.

➤ A warm-up at your own pace.

➤ Periods of hovering (think of short steps).

➤ Hands-free "running" on the stairs.

➤ One-legged stepping.

➤ A well-deserved (and much needed) cooldown.

Because you have the ultimate control of how hard you're working (by increasing or decreasing the level of intensity on the machine), stomp classes are suitable for a variety of fitness levels.

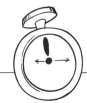

Short Cuts

If you like the idea of stomp classes and your gym hasn't gotten on the bandwagon yet, StairMaster has stomp videotapes that you can use.

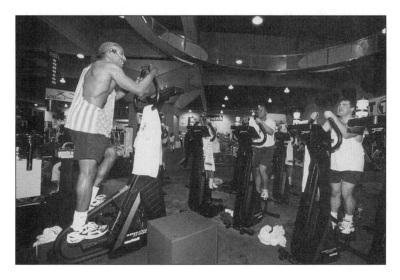

Stomp classes are a great way to make your Stair-Master time productive and fun.

Have Fun

You hear this all the time, so often in fact that it's become a cliché, but if you're not having fun with your exercise you can be reasonably sure you're stepping to the wrong beat. Because your authors are competitive athletes and educated in anatomy and physiology, we're often guilty of getting bogged down in turning exercise into a regimented task instead of what it should be—an expression of your inner joy. Sounds corny, and maybe it is, but go out and chase a Frisbee, ride your mountain bike on a fire road through the woods, body surf at the beach, or do any other of the 10,000 thoroughly delightful physical things you can do and you'll know what we mean. Sure, it's efficient to ride at 72.96 percent of your target zone on the latest state-of-the-art fitness gizmo; however, nothing will get you fitter faster than enjoying yourself.

Ignoring this simple truth is why many of you fail to stick to a fitness regimen even though you know it's good for you. For example, many of the members at Jonathan's gym avoid cardiovascular machines the way kids do brussels sprouts, yet they'll happily go out and play full-court basketball for an hour or two until they're stepping on their tongues. Please don't tell them, but they're getting a great cardiovascular workout—complete with high-intensity intervals. If hoops doesn't do it for you, go to the park, play tennis, toss around a football, take a class in ballroom dancing (it is an Olympic sport), or lace on your blades and go visit a friend. The name of the game is to find physical activities that you enjoy and will do on a consistent basis.

The Least You Need to Know

➤ With an hour almost anything *is* possible.

➤ Whether it's a marathon or a century ride, 60-minute workouts can help get you there.

➤ Classes are a great way to get in shape.

➤ Don't forget to have fun.

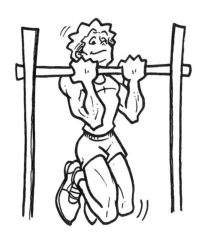

Chapter 18

The Hour of Power

In This Chapter

➤ With an hour, you can meet almost any goal in the weight room

➤ Below the waist or bust

➤ Making a case for above the waist

➤ Splits for the ambitious

Thus far we've made 74 references to the importance of a well-rounded fitness regimen, one that features strength training, cardiovascular work and stretching. Having hammered that point home, we know that some of you have a particular fondness for lifting weights. If heavy metal is your cup of tea, this chapter is for you—virtually no stretching or cardio, just good old pumping iron.

The irony of including a chapter detailing 60-minute strength-training workouts in a book that focuses on short workouts is that unless you're eager to become a bodybuilder, an hour a day is more than enough time to spend in the weight room. Sure, we've read about athletes such as former heavyweight champ Evander Holyfield who was known for doing two- or three-hour strength-training workouts. (Of course, he was making millions of dollars per fight and had a personal trainer who pushed him to exhaustion.) But unless you plan on fighting for the heavyweight title, these marathon-lifting sessions are unnecessary. The plain fact is that you can work all your major muscle groups quite effectively without having your mail and phone calls forwarded to the gym.

The All-in-One Hour

First let's look at a comprehensive, full-body workout that will help you add size and strength. Unlike our previous 60-minute workout, which includes lifting, stretching, and cardio, we aim to incorporate a wider variety and greater quantity of pure strength-training exercises in these workouts. The basic outline of this one-hour-per-day workout is the (ever-essential) quick warm-up and cooldown, 16 exercises, one set each, with two minutes, recovery between sets.

Muscle	Exercise
Legs, hips	Leg press
	Leg extension
	Leg curls
	Standing calf raise
	Seated calf raise
Back	Lat pull downs
	Rows
	Upright row
Chest	Bench press
	Dips
Shoulders	Shoulder press
	Lateral raises
Arms	Seated biceps curl
	Triceps push down
Midsection	Reverse crunch
	Crunch
	Oblique crunch
	Back raise

We like this combination of exercises because it's a good balance between upper body and lower body, and hits all your major muscle groups. Nothing is neglected, yet nothing is overused.

Seated Calf Raise

The only new exercise in this routine is the seated calf raise, which is done on the appropriately named seated calf raise machine. This exercise works the soleus muscle that helps add size and shape to your calves. Here's what you need to know:

1. Sit on the seat with your knees under the kneepads.
2. Position the balls of your feet on the edge of the foot plate.

3. Disengage the brake, allowing your heels to hang over the edge.

4. Rise up onto your toes as high as possible.

5. Return slowly to a position where your heels are hanging down as far as possible to ensure a good stretch.

Seated Calf Raise Tips

Maintain an erect posture; don't rock your trunk back and forth.

Maintain a slow and steady motion throughout the exercise; don't perform it rapidly.

Keep your abdominals tight.

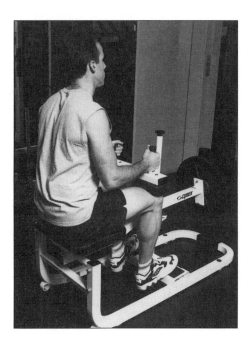

As with the standing calf raise, be sure to get a good stretch in the starting position of the seated calf raise.

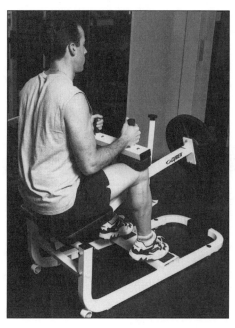

Be sure to come all the way up on your toes at the top of the movement.

Which Way to the Beach?

What if you prefer to place a little extra emphasis on a particular part of your body? Often people want to spend a little extra time and effort on training their upper body. Others favor a lower-body emphasis. To accommodate those of you with a particular bias, here are several programs to help you add a little extra muscle above or below your belt line.

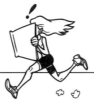

Info to Go

Every gym has them: the turbo-looking guy who has an upper body that resembles a refrigerator and legs that look like they belong to Bambi. While that's taking it to the obvious extreme (one we hope you strenuously avoid), it can be interesting and enjoyable to shake up your typical routine with a slightly different focus. The body is incredibly adaptable and it's often very interesting to experiment and see what happens when you do extra work in one particular area.

The routine listed below will take care of the basics for your legs and abs, and give you plenty of time to work on the body parts above your waist.

Upper-Body Emphasis Routine

Body Part	Exercise
Legs/hips	Leg extension
	Leg curl
Back	Lat pull down
	Row
	Upright row
Chest	Bench press
	Incline press
	Decline press
Shoulders	Military press
	Lateral raise
Arms	Seated dumbbell curl
	Concentration curl
	Triceps push down
	Triceps kickback

Body Part	Exercise
Midsection	Reverse crunch
	Crunch
	Oblique crunch
	Back raise

As you can see, we've kept the leg work to a bare minimum (sorry, we won't get rid of it totally), and added some extra upper-body work, including a couple of more exercises to pump up your arms. This should help stimulate some upper-body muscle mass. Remember, muscle growth doesn't take place instantly, so give it some time—this program should help you do it.

Nice Legs

Perhaps you are that puffed up guy with the buff upper body and the pipe-cleaner legs who has finally come to your senses and wants to balance your disproportionate body. Or maybe you're like Jonathan who has a rather typical competitive cyclist's body—thick thighs and sinewy calves and a muscular, yet slim upper body. In either case, if your muscle-building goals are primarily below your waist, this next program is for you. This program takes care of the basics for your upper body, but really works your lower half.

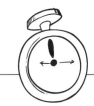

Short Cuts

As we explained in Chapter 6, "Strengthening," we recommend two or three full-body workouts per week. Typically, one set per body part with 10 to 12 reps per set will get the job done—and then some.

Lower–Body Emphasis Routine

Body Part	Exercise
Legs/hips	Squats
	Leg press
	Leg extension
	Leg curl
	Abduction
	Adduction
	Standing calf raise
	Seated calf raise
Back	Lat pull down
	Row
	Upright row

continues

Lower–Body Emphasis Routine   (continued)

Body Part	Exercise
Chest	Bench press
	Dips (assisted if necessary)
Shoulders	Military press
Arms	Biceps curl
	Triceps push down
Midsection	Reverse crunch
	Crunch
	Oblique crunch
	Back raise

Leg work is not fun. Most people dread it because it hurts, but it can have great rewards in terms of both strength and appearance.

Note that while we've emphasized your upper and lower body in these respective workouts, we haven't neglected the other muscles in your body. Furthermore, you'll see that in both the upper- and lower-body routines, we've kept your abdominal work constant. That's because it's important that you not neglect the core muscles of your midsection. Strong abs are the glue that link your upper and lower body. A well-conditioned midsection is essential to core strength and will help prevent lower-back injuries.

Split Personality

Back in Chapter 15, "The 45-Minute Strength-Training Workout," we introduced you to the concept of split routines. A 60-minute split is best suited to those of you who want to pack on some serious muscle.

Push/Pull Split Routine

With the push/pull split, you'll divide your body like this:

➤ Days one and four: legs, back, and biceps.

➤ Days two and five: chest, shoulders, triceps, and midsection.

Days One and Four: Legs, Back, Biceps, and Midsection

Body Part	Exercise
Legs/hips	Leg press
	Leg extension
	Leg curl

Body Part	Exercise
Legs/hips	Abduction
	Adduction
	Standing calf raise
	Seated calf raise
Back	Lat pull down
	Row
	Upright row
	Shrug
Biceps	Seated biceps curl
	Standing barbell curl
	Concentration curl

The only new exercise we introduce in this regimen is the standing biceps curl.

Standing Biceps Curl

This is a classic biceps exercise. If you have back problems, you should do this while standing against a wall. Even if you have a sound back, pay special attention to keeping your back straight and elbows close to your sides.

1. Grip the barbell with palms facing outward, shoulder width apart.
2. Stand with your feet approximately shoulder width apart.
3. Begin with the bar resting on the front of your thighs.
4. Slowly raise the bar by bending your elbows toward your shoulders; slowly lower the bar to the front of your thighs.
5. Control the downward motion during this negative phase.

Standing Biceps Curl Tips

Maintain an erect posture during the entire exercise. Don't use your back to hoist the weight up; if you must do this, the weight is too heavy.

Keep your elbows in close to your sides.

Move throughout your entire range of motion, from elbows straight to fully bent.

Keep your knees slightly bent and your abdominals held tight to protect your back.

213

Keep your arms straight and your knees slightly bent in the start/finish position of the standing biceps curl.

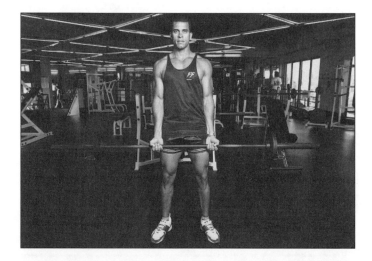

Be sure to keep your back straight and your elbows down as you curl the weight.

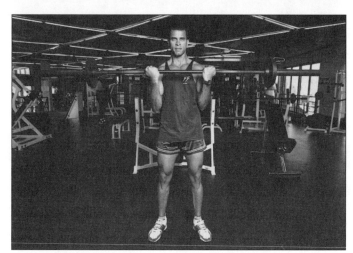

Days Two and Five: Chest, Shoulders, and Triceps

Body Part	Exercise
Chest	Bench press
	Incline press
	Decline press
	Dips
	Flyes
Shoulders	Military press
	Lateral raise

Body Part	Exercise
Shoulders	Front raise
	Reverse flye
Triceps	Triceps push down
	Triceps kickback
	French curls
Midsection	Reverse crunch
	Crunch
	Oblique crunch
	Back raise

We like this split because it gives you a chance to really blast your muscles. In order to keep the amount of sets relatively even from one day to the next, we've included the leg work on the pull day and included your abs and lower back with your pushing exercises. If you do each of these workouts twice per week you'll be in business. Once again, we've added some new exercises.

Front Raises

Front raises are a one-joint exercise, meaning that they isolate the anterior (front) deltoid, the muscle that you use to reach up to grab an apple off a tree. Though you will see people perform the exercise with both arms at the same time, we prefer that you don't. Doing both at the same time will make it easier for you to cheat by dipping your body down as you raise both your arms up.

1. Stand with your feet shoulder width apart.
2. Hold a dumbbell in each hand at your sides with palms facing the legs.
3. Slowly raise one dumbbell up in front of the body until your arm is parallel to the floor.
4. Slowly return to the initial starting position.
5. Do a complete set with one arm before beginning the next arm.

Front Raise Tips

Maintain an erect posture; don't allow your trunk to rock back and forth.

Make sure you don't raise your arm beyond the parallel position.

Keep your abdominals tight.

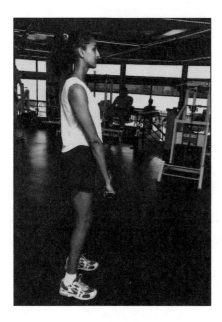 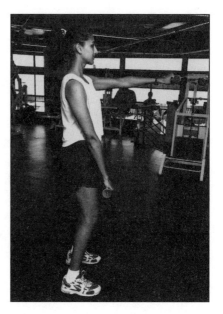

Keep the weight in front of your thigh as you begin the front raise.

Lift the weight until your arm is parallel to the ground.

Reverse Flyes

Reverse flyes are another one-joint exercise that isolates the posterior (rear) deltoid. Again, for the whole muscle to get strong, all of its parts must be worked.

1. Sit on a flat bench and bend forward at the waist.
2. Let the dumbbells hang down at your sides.
3. With a dumbbell in each hand, bring the dumbbells together, palms facing in.
4. Bend your elbows slightly as you raise the dumbbells away from the body.
5. Focus on squeezing your shoulder blades together.
6. With control, return to the starting position.

Reverse Flye Tips

Keep your head facing forward.

Maintain a slow and steady movement throughout the entire exercise.

Make sure the dumbbells don't clang as you bring them together.

Keep your abdominals tight.

Make sure to squeeze your shoulder blades together at the top of the movement.

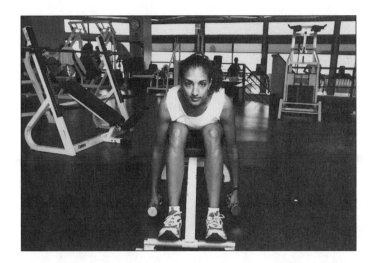

Begin the reverse flye with your arms hanging at your sides.

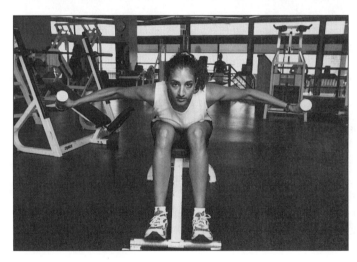

Be sure to keep your torso down and raise your arms until they're parallel to the ground.

French Curls

While this exercise is called the French curl, we don't know why. In any case, it's a great way to isolate and work the triceps muscle.

1. While standing or sitting, raise the dumbbell overhead and bend your elbow to a point where you feel a stretch in the triceps.

2. Straighten your elbow just short of locking it, then slowly return to your initial starting position.

French Curl Tips

Keep your trunk straight; don't shift from side to side in an effort to get the weight up.

Keep your elbow from locking or snapping as you straighten it.

Maintain a slow and steady movement throughout the exercise.

Keep your abdominals tight whether sitting or standing.

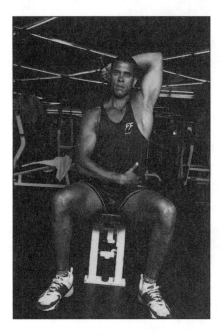

Be sure your torso is straight as you begin the French curl.

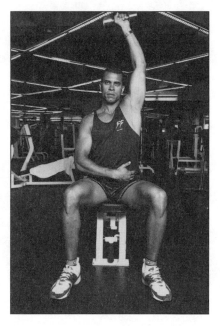

Slowly straighten your elbow, making sure that your upper arm is motionless.

Remember this if you're an aspiring moose: An hour a day three or four times a week is more than sufficient for even the most ambitious lifter or aspiring bodybuilder. The key in the gym should be quality and intensity rather than quantity and volume. Having said all that, we do hope that you lovers of iron will also dedicate some time for stretching and cardio work. Yes, it's great to have a solid, strong, attractive physique to show off at the beach, but to be really fit you'll need to incorporate the other aspect of fitness we've harped on thus far.

The Least You Need to Know

➤ One hour is more than enough time to get a quality workout.

➤ Your routine can emphasize either upper body or lower body; however it is important from an injury point of view to maintain full body balance.

➤ Split routines can give you a chance to concentrate on a select few body parts on each day; however be prepared to commit to more days of exercise.

➤ Lifting may be what you love best, but don't neglect cardio and stretching for a full fitness regimen.

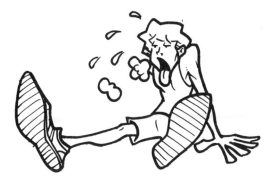

Chapter 19

Don't Waste Your Time

In This Chapter

➤ Right makes might

➤ Some stretches can be harmful

➤ Exercises to avoid

➤ Forget feeling the burn

Joe's grandfather, who lived to the advanced age of 94 without ever exercising or eating a green vegetable (save for pickles), thought anything more strenuous than watching a horse race or playing cards was a waste of time. Considering his age and health, he was hard to argue with. However, most people under the age of 94 know the reasons for working out—stress reduction, looking good, feeling good, injury prevention, improved sports performance, and more. That said, there's nothing worse than a well-intentioned trip to the gym that doesn't produce any results, or worse, causes an injury.

Unfortunately, we see it all the time. Virtually every time we're in a gym, we see people doing exercises that we'd categorize as dopey, dangerous, and/or useless. Often the culprit is bad (okay, horrible) form, which clearly compromises the safety and effectiveness of the exercise.

Since we prefer that you learn from us rather than from an "expert" weaned on back issues of *Muscle & Fitness*, in this chapter we'll highlight some of the most common mistakes made in the gym. After all, a workout, even a short one, that leaves you hobbling around is not exactly a wise choice.

Cardio No-No's

Pick up a book on running and you might think that logging a good cardiovascular workout is only slightly less complicated than nuclear fusion. To state the obvious, doing your cardiovascular (CV) workout shouldn't be that tricky—especially if you follow the guidelines we laid out for you in Chapter 5, "Aerobics." While it isn't rocket science, there are a few pitfalls you should avoid. Here are a couple of the most common CV abuses.

Cheating on the StairMaster

Cheating on the StairMaster by hanging on the handrails makes the caloric expenditure readout inaccurate and places undue stress on your elbows and wrists. In addition, it does nothing to help your workout. If you must, hold the rails lightly, stand up straight, and then have at it. Odds are that you won't be cranking at the highest level for 30 minutes at a pop.

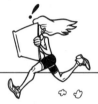

Info to Go

Jonathan was coaching a woman who couldn't lose weight despite the fact that she worked out every day with the StairMaster set on the top level for 30 minutes. (To put this in context, Jonathan once trained a gifted triathlete, a 2:40 marathoner, one of the few people he ever saw max out on the StairMaster during a 30-minute workout.) While this woman was a reasonably fit 40-something, she couldn't run a sub–three-hour marathon to save a rain forest. The difference was good form. When Jonathan checked her out on the StairMaster, she grabbed the handrails, locked her elbows, and fluttered her feet as if she were stomping grapes. The locked-elbows approach is a bit like gently stepping on a scale while hanging from a chinning bar.

Holding On for Dear Life

Just as cheating on a StairMaster can jeopardize a good workout, the same is true of holding onto a treadmill. Obviously, you should use the handrail of the treadmill for stability if you need it, but all too often we see folks holding on for dear life as they walk up a steep grade. If their hands ever slipped, they'd fly off the back of the thing.

Instead, you're better off decreasing the grade and/or speed and striding along with your arms swinging, or holding on loosely if necessary for balance.

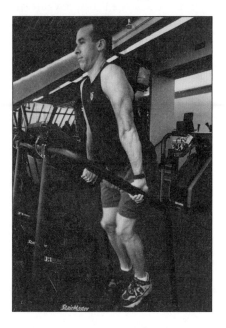

Jonathan demonstrating atrocious, but not uncommon, form.

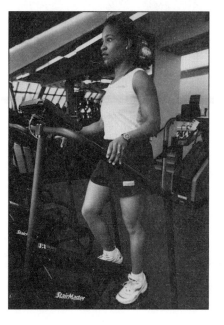

Here's Deidre doing everything right.

Hang Loose

Throughout the book we've reminded you about the key elements of stretching: Don't bounce, hold your stretch for 20 to 30 seconds, and don't push to the point of pain. If you remember those guidelines, you've avoided the most common stretching pitfalls. However, there are several common stretches that we'd like to see you skip.

Standing Toe Touch

Yes, it's one of the most common stretches out there. Look at the starting line of your local 10K race and you'll see half the field doing it. The standing toe touch is a great stretch for your hamstrings; however, it can place too much stress on your lower back. Since there's an equally effective alternative, it's better to do a seated hamstring stretch (pictured on next page). If you prefer to

Stop Short

The standing toe touch is especially dangerous for those of you with back problems, particularly herniated or bulging discs.

223

remain standing for practical reasons, stretching one leg at a time while supporting your back is preferable. To do this, bend one knee about 30° and place your hands on it as you extend your other leg in front; you'll feel the stretch in your hamstring.

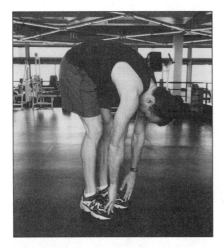

The standing toe touch is as common as sweat in the gym.

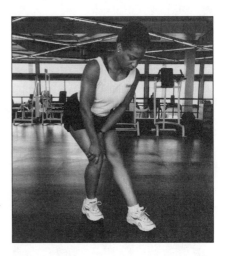

This alternative standing hamstring stretch takes the stress off your lower back.

Hurdler's Stretch

The hurdler's stretch is another gym favorite that we'd like to see go the way of the dodo. It's a great way to stretch your hamstrings, but by bending the opposite knee back like a hurdler in midflight, you're placing undue stress on the connective tissue of the bent knee. By simply tucking the knee in the other way, with the foot touching the inner thigh of the opposite leg, you'll protect your knee while still getting the same stretch for your hamstrings.

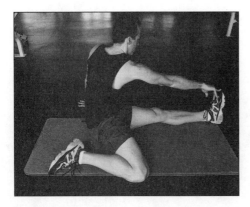

Jonathan's knees are not happy in this position.

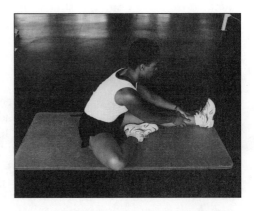

Deidre's knees are safe in this stretch.

Yoga Plough

We're big proponents of yoga. And there's no better way to learn this ancient art than by taking a class taught by a qualified teacher. What makes us nervous is when we see someone who's hardly warmed up, doing one of the classic yoga stretches called the plough pose. (Halasana to you yoga-philes.) The plough requires that you lie on your back. Next you raise your legs, hips, and buttocks off the ground you let your feet lower to the floor behind your head, keeping your legs straight.

While the plough is a great way to stretch your neck and back, it also puts way too much stress on your cervical spine, the section of your spine in your neck. The cervical section of your spine is not designed to bear weight, and doing so risks serious injury. We're not suggesting that everyone who does the plough is going to get hurt, and yes, we know of people who've done this pose for years without incident. Still, we'd prefer that you modify the plough so that your knees don't go past your shoulders. You can also just pull your bent knees back to your chest.

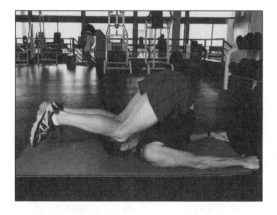

The yoga plough places unnecessary stress on the cervical spine.

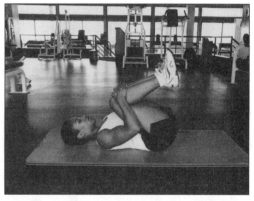

This variation stretches your lower back while protecting your neck.

Strength

If you're scouting for bad form, there's no better place to find it than the weight room. All too often, lifters worry about doing as many reps as possible or moving as much weight as possible at the expense of form. Keep in mind that you're in the weight room to gain strength, not demonstrate it.

Bad Crunch Form

Most of us want flat, athletic-looking abs—did anyone say Olympic sprinter Marion Jones?—and most of us are willing to work to get them. Often, however, people think that to get this GI Joe look they have to pound hundreds of sit-ups a day. Very often when Jonathan meets with a new member of his gym, he runs into know-it-all types who think of his services as a waste of their time. "Heck," said a guy we'll call Mr. Abs, "I do 500 crunches a day."

Fine and dandy except for one massive drawback: If you're doing 500 crunches at a time, we can wager a small townhouse that your form stinks. Case in point: When Jonathan asked Mr. Abs to do a few crunches, this very ambitious fellow proceeded with textbook bad form. Not only was he jerking his head forward like a famished woodpecker, he was barely getting his shoulders off the mat, holding his breath, and arching his back to boot. (Other than that he was perfect.) When Jonathan corrected his form, Mr. Abs was barely able to complete a set of 10.

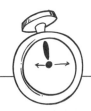

Short Cuts

Making sure you use sound technique when you work out will get you fitter faster, with less chance of injury.

Forget the Jane Fonda "feel the burn" mentality. The burning sensation absolutely does not mean that you're burning fat around your abdominal muscles—it's just a sign of lactic acid accumulation.

Good Crunch Form

Here's what you should keep in mind when you do your crunches: Slowly curl forward for three seconds up to an angle of about 30°, pause, and slowly lower yourself back to the starting position. Be sure to keep your lower back pressed into the floor at all times and keep your hands lightly clasped behind your head, with your elbows wide, rather than tucked in front of you. Be sure to exhale on the way up and inhale on the return.

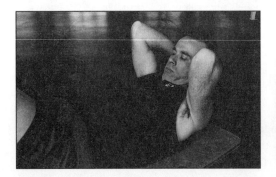

The most common crunch mistakes are tucking your chin, using limited range of motion, and moving too fast.

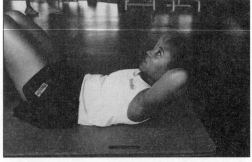

Imagine a tennis ball between your chin and your chest as you do your crunches.

Exploding Myths

If you ever want to hear an exercise psychologist rant and rave for an hour or so, just ask Jonathan what he thinks about *lifting explosively.*

We'll spare you the physics lecture, but by lifting fast, you're putting much more stress on your connective tissue and greatly increasing your chance of injury. Furthermore, you're introducing momentum into the equation and making the exercise much easier. When Deidre lifted competitively, her goal was to demonstrate strength. To achieve her aim, she used every trick in the book to help move the weight. Lifting fast was one such trick. Now that she's no longer competing (she was frequently injured), her goal in the weight room is to stay strong and healthy. Since she doesn't really care how much weight she moves, she pays strict attention to her technique. By adhering to the three seconds up, three seconds down cadence—with a slight pause in between—she ensures maximum results and minimum risk.

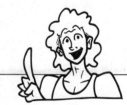

Workout Words

Lifting explosively is the practice of lifting the weight as fast as possible, in a misguided attempt to improve your speed or power. Why the objection? Well, just that it's not safe and it's not effective.

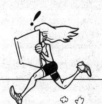

Info to Go

The one possible exception to the don't-lift-explosively rule comes into play with an exercise like the power clean, which can only be performed explosively. While some strength coaches consider this a staple of an athlete's training program, many professional strength coaches (including us) consider the orthopedic risks of the power clean far too great for anyone except an Olympic weight lifter.

Double Leg Lift with Straight Legs

Where do we start? The part about them not doing any good or the part about them being dangerous? Much like the full sit-up, this exercise doesn't work your abs effectively because your hip flexors produce the movement. Adding injury to insult, they place a tremendous stress on your lower back.

A far better option is reverse curls. While far less impressive looking than leg lifts, this exercise is a safe way to work your lower abs. Keep the movement small and keep your lower back pressed into the mat at all times. Lift your tailbone a few inches off the floor, pause at the top, and slowly return to the starting position. To make sure that you get the most out of the exercise, be sure to exhale as you lift and inhale as you lower.

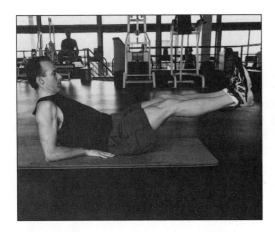

Leave the double leg lifts back in high school gym class.

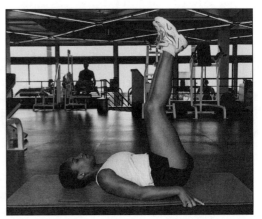

The reverse crunch requires only a small, but challenging movement.

Bad Bench Press Form

The oh-too-common question, "How much do you bench?" is one of the most dangerous and counterproductive things you'll ever hear in the gym. Listen carefully, men, because most often you're the culprits. Too often, egos get in the way in the weight room and the focus shifts from the goal of gaining strength to the goal of showing off. (If you ever want to see the result of the "Fragile Male Ego Syndrome," watch what happens when our petite little 130-pound Deidre walks into the weight room and bangs out perfect reps with 135 pounds. It's amazing how quickly guys will pile the weight on with no regard for their safety in an attempt to avoid being shown up by "a girl.")

The most common mistakes in this classic lift are

➤ Arching the back.

➤ Holding the breath.

➤ Lowering the bar too fast.

➤ Bouncing the bar off your chest.

Yes, this makes it a lot easier to impress your friends, but all too often the result of bad bench press form is a shoulder, wrist, or back injury.

While on the topic of things not to do on the bench press, our other pet peeve is loading the bar up to test your one rep max (1RM). While seeing how much weight you can do for one rep is a standard benchmark used by fitness enthusiasts, it's a better way to blow out your shoulder, tear your pec, or bruise your sternum—all of which we've seen happen to poor slobs attempting a maximal bench press. If you want to mark your progress, test your 10RM (the most weight you can press for 10 reps) every once in a while.

Proper bench press form means keeping your knees bent and your feet flat on the floor at all times. If your back arches off of the bench in this position, place your feet to the bench or use 45-pound plates as risers. Slowly lift and lower the bar—three seconds in each direction, pause for a split second at your chest; never bounce the bar. Exhale on the way up and inhale on the way down. Last but not least, always use a spotter. If one isn't available, use a machine or dumbbells.

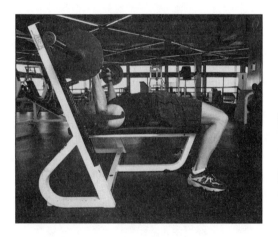

Jonathan couldn't have worse form if he tried—arched back, no spotter, no collars on the bar.

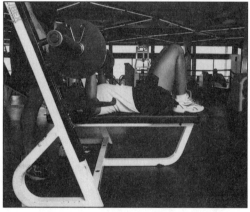

Deidre demonstrates her usual pristine form.

Some More No-No's

Sometimes our objections are to good exercises done with poor form. Other times we simply don't like the exercise itself.

Barbell Bent Rows, Good Mornings, and Stiff-Legged Dead Lifts

You can execute these three exercises with perfect form and we still won't like them. Here's why. Think of how you're always told to lift things: bend at the knees, not at the back. (Deidre spends half her professional life teaching back patients how to use the big muscles of their legs rather than their back muscles when they lift.)

To us students of anatomy, bending forward at the waist without supporting your back is known as "unsupported forward flexion." Whatever it's called, it can wreak havoc on your back. During these exercises not only are you performing unsupported forward flexion (which is why we don't recommend the standing toe touch), but you're doing it with added weight, which makes it that much more unsafe for your back. While we're not saying that you'll get hurt if you dare to try these exercises, why take the risk? Since there are safer alternatives to these exercises, there's really no reason to do them. Here are some alternatives.

Instead of doing bent rows with a barbell, use a dumbbell while supporting your back by placing your other arm and leg on a bench. It's just as effective for your back muscles, and much safer.

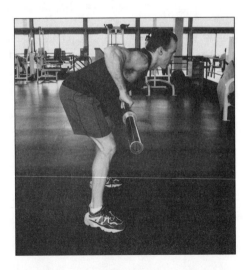

Bending forward at your waist with no support can be dangerous for your back.

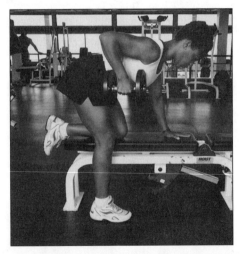

By supporting your back on the bench, you get the same benefits without the risk.

Good mornings and stiff-legged dead lifts are a physical therapist's dream. Ask Deidre: They keep her in business. The idea of both is to strengthen the lower back. In the case of stiff-legged dead lifts, there are those who suggest that your hamstrings are strengthened as well. (But that's another argument.)

Instead, why not do back raises on a mat or bench? They are much safer and just as effective. Move slowly through the range of motion and give a little pause at the top.

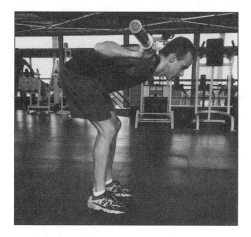

Good mornings are a chiropractor's best friend.

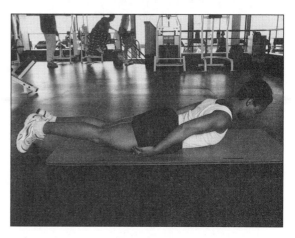

Back raises on the mat are far safer than good mornings.

A Zillion Leg Lifts

Another exercise error that drives us to drink unfiltered water is seeing people doing countless leg lifts in an attempt to "slim" and "tone" their thighs. (Women are the big culprits here.) Here's the scoop. That burning sensation you feel by the end of the set has nothing to do with burning fat in that area. That's because if you work a muscle hard enough, it will grow, not shrink. If you choose a weight that lets you do hundreds of reps, it's not enough stimulus to cause any growth, but it's sure not going to make anything shrink. Considering why most people torture themselves with this exercise, it's a waste of time. If you want to slim down, we prefer you practice this simple formula: Consume fewer calories than you burn. The time you spend doing those leg lifts is much better spent doing some cardio work and burning some calories.

Full Sit-Ups

While we've already criticized your high school phys ed teacher for a number of exercise sins, let's look at one more. What's wrong with sit-ups? We hate to sound like a broken record, but it's the usual: They're not safe and they're not effective.

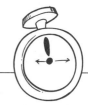

Short Cuts

The best replacement for sit-ups is crunches. Please note that there's no need to go beyond about 30° on the way up. Refer to Chapter 10, "The 15-Minute Strength-Training Workout," for a rundown of proper crunch form.

Here's why. When you anchor your feet (by having someone hold them down or placing them under a desk), the muscles in the front of your hips (known as your hip flexors) help to pull you up. If your hip flexors are working, it means that your abdominal muscles aren't doing the lion's share of the work. In addition, bringing those nasty hip flexors into the equation, you place undue stress on your lower back.

Arching Back for Biceps Curls

Second in line to the bench press for exercises that cause testosterone to fly are biceps curls. For a variety of reasons, our culture adores big biceps, which is why guys often let their egos get in the way. The most common error with guys who try and hoist as much as they can is arching their back and throwing their pelvis forward. Sure it makes it easier, but again, it jeopardizes the well-being of your back.

Here's what you need to remember: Keep your shoulders over your hips and your hips over your ankles. Don't let your elbows raise during the exercise—that involves your shoulders and does your biceps no good.

Sorry guys, if you've been cheating, you'll most likely need to decrease the weight you're using, but you'll find the exercise far more effective.

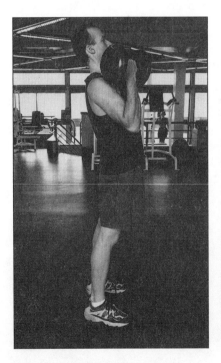

Note the locked knees, high elbows, and backward-leaning posture.

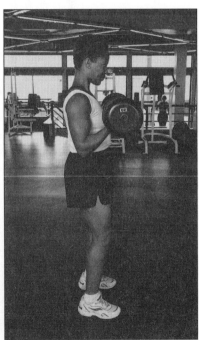

Keep your knees slightly bent and your back straight as you do your curls.

While this is far from an exhaustive list of mistakes made in the gym—we didn't mention sleeping in the sauna or running backward on the treadmill—they are some of the most common. We hope this chapter will help you to avoid some of those pitfalls and keep your exercise time safe and productive.

The Least You Need to Know

➤ Make the most of your time by performing exercises correctly; you'll see results more readily.

➤ While you may feel strong by lifting more weight, doing so incorrectly will cause you more harm than good.

➤ Doing 100 reps when you can do 10 is a waste of time.

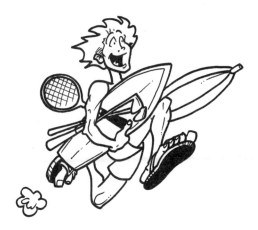

Chapter 20

Weekend Warrior—Conditioning for Sports

In This Chapter

➤ Strength-training for your sport

➤ Elite athletes or weekend warriors both need flexibility

➤ Sports specific training routines to help your game

Thus far we've devoted considerable space to telling you about the countless benefits of working out. Between improving your health, injury prevention, and just plain old looking good you can't afford *not* to exercise. We hope we've been preaching to the converted, but there's another great reason to work out: to improve your performance in your favorite sport. Whether it be swimming, skiing, martial arts, or badminton, cross-training will make you a more potent athlete.

Since our focus is on short workouts, we're assuming that you're not planning to swim the English Channel or become a professional wrestler. However, that's no reason to think sports specific training won't help you immensely as a weekend warrior. There's a reason that virtually every committed athlete, from tennis players to jockeys, does some form of strength training. Of course, different sports demand a different conditioning regimen.

In this chapter we'll outline cardiovascular, strength, and stretching workouts specifically designed for your sport. Our aim, of course, is to make sure these workouts will fit into your busy schedule.

Running

Whether your goal is to finish a 5K or 10K road race, a half marathon, or a full marathon, there are a variety of things you can do in the gym to help you run faster and healthier. Obviously, the best way to improve your cardio fitness for running is to run. When running isn't practical (or if you're feeling leg weary), there are a variety of ways to cross-train in the gym.

We like the newfangled elliptical trainers that are popping up in gyms from coast to coast. A mixture of a cross-country ski machine and StairMaster, this low-impact machine allows you to work your upper body by pumping the handholds (ski poles basically) and your legs without any of the pounding you get from jogging.

The NordicTrack, the most commonly found cross-country ski simulators in most gyms, has long been a favorite of runners. (In fact, cross-country skiing on real snow may be the best cross-training sport for all sports.) Like the elliptical trainer, the NordicTrack provides a nonimpact cardio workout. While you can get a great workout on this machine, getting comfortable with the balance on the NordicTrack takes a bit of patience.

If those machines don't do it for you, cycling—indoors or out—is a good way to build leg strength and cardiovascular fitness while eliminating the pounding of running. Experiment with riding out of the saddle for a few minutes at a time. It helps stretch your legs, really works your quadriceps, and elevates your heart rate.

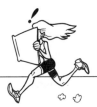

Info to Go

Another great cross-training workout for runners is to do a minitriathlon in the gym. Start, for example, on the stationary bike. Warm up for 10 minutes and then speed up to roughly 70 percent effort for five additional minutes. Hop on the elliptical trainer for 15 minutes at 70 percent and, if you have the time and/or the energy, finish off with 15 minutes on another cardio machine of your choice. (We love the Concept II rowing machine.) Not only does this reduce the tedium of hammering away on one machine, you'll work up a terrific sweat, burn plenty of calories, and give your runner's legs a blessed rest.

What about strength training for a sport that relies on the legs? While the runner with the strongest muscles doesn't always win the race, the one with the weakest muscles often doesn't even make it to the starting line. That's because runners who do nothing but run are often tight as a drum and hence often hurt. Don't worry about the myth that lifting weights will bulk you up and slow you down. On the contrary, lifting will help restore muscular symmetry and help you sidestep common running injuries such as tendinitis, bursitis, and hamstring strains.

Here's a sample 30-minute strength-training program for runners. Do one set of each exercise for sets of 10 to 12 reps, two or three times per week. Remember: Slow controlled movements—three seconds up, three seconds down, with one-minute recovery between exercises.

Body Part	Exercises
Legs/hips	Leg press
	Leg curl
	Abduction
	Adduction
	Standing calf raise
	Seated calf raise
Back	Lat pull down or pull-ups (assisted if necessary to complete 10 good reps)
Chest	Dips (assisted if necessary) or bench press
Shoulders	Shoulder press
Arms	Seated biceps curl
	Triceps push down
Midsection	Reverse crunches
	Crunches
	Obliques
	Back raises

Unless you weigh as much as a feather-light Kenyan marathoner or run on soft trails, stretching is of the utmost important for runners since the repetitive motion shortens the muscles in your legs and back. This program doesn't take long to do and once you feel the difference you'll be glad you did it.

Body Part	Stretch
Lower back	The spinal twist/lower back and hip stretch
Hip flexors	Lunge stretch
Quadriceps	Standing quadriceps stretch
Hamstrings	Sitting hamstring stretch
Calves	Gastrocnemius
	Standing gastrocnemius stretch
Soleus	Standing soleus stretch

Cycling

Cycling is many things to many people. Some want to race, others may want to tour through the countryside on the weekend. If you're an off-road enthusiast, you'll be storming down trails on a knobby-tired mountain bike. (You may want to do all three.) In any case, an overall conditioning program will have you riding more miles with greater ease.

Again, the best way to improve your riding is to ride. During the week, try to go for a spin on your bike—even if it's only for 30 minutes. (If you're riding indoors on a stationary bike, 20 minute will do.) Don't worry about tales of two- and three-hour rides through the mountains; the key is to try and ride as much as your schedule allows. Try and use your bike for transportation. Whenever possible, ride outdoors. The difference between 30 minutes on a Lifecycle indoors or in a *spin class* and watching the world zip by outside is the difference between a TV dinner and a fine French meal.

If you are a fair-weather rider who wants to get the most out of your cycling time, there's a great indoor trainer called the Compu Trainer that allows you to ride your own bike through a variety of simulated courses. Jonathan uses it extensively and not only because of his antisocial nature. It's a great time saver—no need to bundle up in the cold, no changing flats, and no fighting traffic—just put your head down and go.

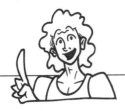

Workout Words

Spin class is an indoor group class geared toward cycling. The bikes are specially designed to provide variable levels of resistance and don't allow you to coast.

The Compu Trainer eliminates any weather-related excuses for cyclists.

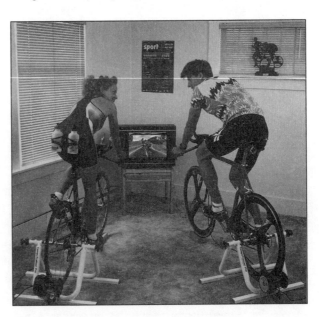

Cyclists can benefit greatly (in terms of both improved performance and decreased risk of injury) from the increased strength gained from a couple of sessions in the weight room each week. Here's a lifting program for you two-wheel fans. Aim for two or three sessions per week and sets of 10 to 12 repetitions.

Body Part	Exercises
Legs/hips	Squat or leg press
	Leg extension
	Leg curl
Back	Lat pull downs or pull-ups
	Upright rows
Chest	Dips or bench press
Shoulders	Military press
Arms	Seated biceps curl
	Triceps push down
Midsection	Reverse crunches
	Crunches
	Oblique crunches
	Back raises

Anyone who has ridden a racing bike knows that cyclists spend their time in a flexed posture. This tends to cause tightness in the hip flexors, pectorals, and neck extensors. Try the following stretches to combat the bent-over-bike syndrome.

Body Part	Stretch
Hip flexors	Lunge
Quadriceps	Standing quadriceps stretch
Hamstrings	Sitting hamstring stretch
Calves	Standing gastrocnemius/soleus stretch
Pectorals	Pectoral stretch

Tennis

Back in the '80s, Martina Navratilova began lifting weights and blowing her opponents off the court. In the '90s, Andre Aggassi got serious, hit the weight room, and began winning grand slams. More recently, if you have any doubts about the need for an overall conditioning program for tennis players, look at the Williams sisters—Venus and Serena—and their sculpted bodies.

A complete training program for tennis includes the big three: cardio work, strength training, and stretching. Cardio cross-training will help your overall conditioning so that you're able to hang in there during long rallies and at the end of a tough match. Unless you plan on challenging the club pro to a three-set winner-take-all match, 20 or 30 minutes of aerobic activity should be enough. Flip back to Chapter 11, "The 30-Minute Cardio Workout," for more on cross-training.

Try alternating running for one or two training sessions per week. If you want to spare your legs (or you don't like running) use the StairMaster or Lifecycle and set it on one of the interval programs. If you have the time, do one or two steady, moderately paced workouts in addition.

A good strength program can not only help your overall game—"Hey, Herb, what did you do to your serve?"—but can keep the dreaded "tennis elbow" (lateral epicondylitis for those of you scoring at home) at bay. Try this short routine two or three times per week, 10 to 12 repetitions per set.

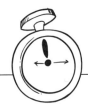

Short Cuts

Clearly, tennis is a game of stops and starts—between points, games, and sets. As a result, interval training—versus steady continuous training—will more closely simulate the cardiovascular demands of a singles match.

Body Part	Exercise
Legs/hips	Lunges
	Adduction
	Abduction
Back	Rows
Chest	Bench press
Shoulders	Military press
Arms	Seated biceps curl
	Triceps extension
	Wrist curls
Midsection	Crunch
	Reverse crunch
	Rotary torso
	Back raise

Tennis is a game that requires ample doses of lunging, sprinting, and reaching. Ask any weekend warrior who plays a lot of singles and they'll regale you with tales of strained or pulled hamstring muscles or back muscles. And unless you play on a forgiving surface like clay, hard courts are tough on your knees. The stretches below should help combat the pounding that a hard game of singles doles out. Try them before a match as well as in the gym.

Body Part	Exercise
Pectorals	Pectoral stretch
Lower back	Spinal twist/lower back and hip stretch
Adductors	Groin stretch
Quadriceps	Standing quadriceps stretch
Hamstrings	Sitting hamstrings stretch
Calves	Standing gastrocnemius/soleus stretch

Because tennis is such a game of technique and timing, your conditioning program must leave you time to whack those furry little yellow balls!

Golf

Okay, stop chuckling. Perhaps you won't find John Daly going toe to toe with the football players at the superstars competition, but a solid conditioning program can help improve your performance on the links.

No, the cardiovascular demands of walking a golf course don't exactly match those of running a marathon, but it can be tiring by the end of the day. Any basic cardiovascular training such as jogging or brisk walking, cycling, or any of the many other pieces of equipment in the gym will help you keep your weight down and build your endurance. If you can do 20 to 30 minutes of training three times a week, you'll be stronger with the driver late in the day.

Most professional golfers don't look as if they've lost any sleep overdoing it in the weight room. However, since Tiger Woods's ascendancy to the top of the sport (and perhaps the best ever), more and more linksters have followed Woods's example and hit the weight room. Dr. Wayne Westcott, fitness and research director at the South Shore YMCA in Quincy, Massachusetts, has done extensive research to show that a basic strength-training program can significantly improve your club speed, which directly translates to increased driving distance.

Try the exercises listed below twice a week. They should help get you strong and leave you plenty of time for the greens.

Body Part	Exercise
Legs/hips	Leg press
	Leg curl
Back	Lat pull down
Chest	Bench press

continues

continued

Body Part	Exercise
Shoulders	Military press
Arms	Seated biceps curl
	Triceps push down
	Wrist curl
Midsection	Reverse crunches
	Crunches
	Rotary torso
	Back raise

In case you haven't noticed, swinging a golf club can cause a great deal of stress to your back and hips. Here are some stretches to help you avoid injuries.

Body Part	Stretch
Pectorals	Pectoral stretch
Lower back/hips	Spinal twist/lower back and hip stretch
Quadriceps	Quadriceps stretch
Hamstrings	Hamstring stretch
Calves	Standing gastrocnemius/soleus stretch

Skating

Whether it's ice-skating or in-line skating, skating requires significant leg strength and, if you're skating on hilly terrain, places a hefty demand on your cardiovascular system.

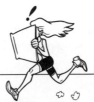

Info to Go

A while back, Nautilus (among others) introduced skating simulators for the gym. Unfortunately, they were awkward and never caught on. Plus, it wasn't nearly as much fun as the real thing, although your feet didn't get cold.

To repeat: If you want to improve your skating, it's best to skate whenever you can. When you can't lace 'em up, cycling (including the stationary bike) is good cross-training. (Olympians like Eric Heiden have competed at elite levels in both sports because of the similarity of the two activities.)

A skaters' strength program should emphasize the leg muscles. However, building up your abdominal and lower-back muscles should be emphasized because they help you maintain your aerodynamic tuck and avoid soreness and injury. These exercises should be performed two or three times a week, 10 to 12 repetitions per set.

Body Part	Exercise
Legs/hips	Leg press or squat
	Lunge
	Abduction
	Adduction
Back	Lat pull down
Chest	Bench press
Shoulders	Military press
Arms	Seated biceps curl
	Triceps push down
	Wrist curl
Midsection	Reverse crunches
	Crunches
	Rotary torso
	Back raise

The following stretching routine at each gym workout and before and after you skate will keep you limber and (we hope) injury free. In addition, increased flexibility usually translates into more speed. (You'll probably find them easier if you don't have your skates on, unless you have exemplary balance and grace.)

Body Part	Exercise
Neck extensors	Neck extensor stretch
Pectorals	Pectoral stretch
Lower back	Spinal twist/lower back and hip stretch
Hip flexors	Lunges
Quadriceps	Standing quadriceps stretch
Hamstrings	Sitting hamstring stretch
Calves	Standing gastrocnemius/soleus stretch

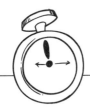

Short Cuts

Before hitting the slopes, virtually any cardiovascular training will do. The idea is to improve your overall conditioning and, if necessary, control your weight. Aim for three cardio sessions per week for 20 to 30 minutes in your target zone.

Skiing/Snowboarding

Skiing and snowboarding are high on the list of "classic" weekend warrior sports. Think of the enthusiast who's largely inactive but signs on for a ski trip with friends. By the end of the weekend, our psyched snow bunny has busted his butt on the slopes so many times he's barely able to get out of a chair. Don't let us dampen your enthusiasm. Both these activities can be tons of fun, but they are also very stressful on someone without the requisite conditioning. Do a bit of prep work in the gym and you can make your time on the slopes safer and more enjoyable.

Try to do the following strength-training exercises two or three times per week. They'll help your balance and overall stamina. We can't guarantee that you'll shred the slopes with any more grace (lessons are best here), but they will help you avoid injury and that postexercise soreness.

Body Part	Exercise
Legs/hips	Leg press
	Lunges
	Leg curl
Back	Lat pull down
Chest	Bench press
Shoulders	Military press
Arms	Seated biceps curl
	Triceps push down
Midsection	Reverse crunches
	Crunches
	Rotary torso
	Back raise

Just because you're out with your buddies, don't forget to stretch. Since we can safely assume that it's cold wherever you'll ski, remember what we said back in Chapter 7, "Start with Stretching." Stretching cold muscles requires extra care in order to avoid injury. Do these stretches during your regular workouts and before you hit the slopes. Try to warm up a little before you stretch and be sure to stretch gently.

Body Part	Stretch
Lower back	Spinal twist/lower back and hip stretch
Hip flexors	Lunges
Quadriceps	Standing quadriceps stretch
Hamstrings	Sitting hamstring stretch
Calves	Standing gastrocnemius/soleus stretch

Martial Arts

In the martial arts, the old adage of "it's better to give than receive" is especially true. However, before you're doling it out on a regular basis, you'll do plenty of receiving. Strength training won't improve your skills in the dojo (martial arts school), but it will help soften the blows.

Most bouts in the martial arts involve two or three minutes of intense exertion followed by a rest. As a result, it's not necessary to do long cardiovascular workouts once you've established a basic level of fitness. (If you're just starting out, don't head to the nearest track and start sprinting.)

Interval training that involves hard efforts for two or three minutes followed by a short recovery period will prepare your cardiovascular system for the task at hand (or leg). For example, you could run up a hill for three minutes at a challenging pace and walk down to recover. (Using the incline feature on the treadmill does much the same thing.) Repeat this four-minute grouping four or five times.

You can also do intervals on a stationary bike. Set the resistance higher than you can comfortably pedal when you're sitting down, stand out of the saddle, and hammer away for three minutes. Sit and cycle easily for a minute to calm your racing heart. Again, aim for four or five repetitions.

There are always Tae-Bo and other kickboxing classes offered at the gym. While they certainly won't teach you martial arts, they're good ways to prepare your body for a more intense martial arts regimen.

Most advanced martial artists lift weights. Here's a short routine you can do two or three times a week to ready you for the rigors ahead.

Body Part	Exercise
Legs/hips	Leg press
	Leg curl
	Abduction
	Adduction
Back	Rows or pull-ups

continues

continued

Body Part	Exercise
Chest	Bench press or dips
Shoulders	Military press
Arms	Seated biceps curl
	Triceps kickback
Midsection	Midsection reverse crunches
	Crunches
	Rotary torso
	Back raise

Flexibility is a big part of virtually every discipline that we know of in the martial arts. While you're likely to do plenty of strength training in class, it's a good idea to show up limber. Here are some stretches to keep you failing away.

Body Part	Stretch
Pectorals	Pectoral stretch
Lower back	Spinal twist/lower back and hip stretch
Hip flexors	Lunge
Adductors	Groin stretch
Hamstrings	Sitting hamstring stretch
Quadriceps	Standing quadriceps stretch
Calves	Standing gastrocnemius/soleus stretch

Paddling

Watch any SUV ad these days and odds are someone is paddling a kayak down a raging river. Even if paddling raging white water isn't your thing, the fact is that canoeing and kayaking are great ways to get and stay in shape as well as experience one of Mother Nature's most profound teachers: water. For people who truly loathe lifting weights, paddling allows you to build up your upper body much the way walking or running works your legs.

Initially when you start paddling a canoe or kayak, the biggest challenge is learning proper technique and becoming comfortable in a new medium. In other words, the cardiovascular demands will not be that great. Once you get more comfortable out there, the best way to improve your power is to do any aerobic activity that elevates your heart rate to 70 percent or more. (Running, cycling, and cross-country skiing are all excellent—indoors or out.)

Even though we just said that paddling is a great way to improve your upper body strength without lifting weights, the plain facts are that if you want to improve as a paddler, punching the clock in the gym is the best way that we know. Joe, a two-time member of the U.S. National Marathon Kayak team, would rather paddle than lift virtually any day, but pumps plenty of iron because he knows how much better he'll perform in the boat. In addition, strength training can minimize the amount of paddle-related injuries to your lower back and shoulders.

Body Part	Exercise
Legs/hips	Leg extension
	Leg curl
Back	Pull-ups (assisted if necessary)
	Rows
Chest	Bench press
	Dips (assisted if necessary)
Shoulders	Military press
	Lateral raise
Arms	Seated biceps curl
	Triceps push down
Midsection	Reverse crunch
	Crunch
	Rotary torso
	Back raise

If you log serious paddle time you'll need to stretch, since sitting in a narrow kayak can leave your legs and lower back tight and, for those who are chronically tight, numb. Do the following and you should experience happy paddling.

Body Part	Exercise
Pectorals	Pectoral stretch
Lower back	Spinal twist/lower back and hip stretch
Hip flexors	Lunge
Quadriceps	Standing quadriceps stretch
Hamstrings	Sitting hamstring stretch
Calves	Standing gastrocnemius/soleus stretch

The Least You Need to Know

➤ A comprehensive fitness regimen requires stretching so your muscles remain flexible and you remain injury free.

➤ Choose your sport and do the recommended stretches and exercises.

➤ Stretching and exercising will improve your performance in your chosen sport.

➤ A stretching regimen of as little as five minutes per day is enough to provide you with the flexibility your body needs.

Part 5

Away from the Gym

In a perfect world, you'd get to the gym whenever you want. Since that's not always the case, it's time to look at how to stay in shape away from the gym.

In this part, we'll provide you with strategies for exercising when you're out of town on business or pleasure. If you're stuck at the office, you'll find lots of tips for squeezing in a workout at your desk.

Appropriate and comfortable clothes and footwear will help make your workout safe and enjoyable and make you look good. Finally, you'll find tips for safely and effectively participating in a variety of activities in hot or cold conditions.

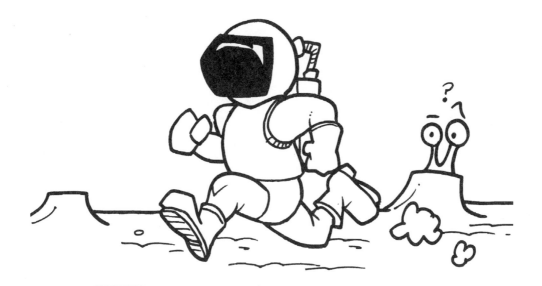

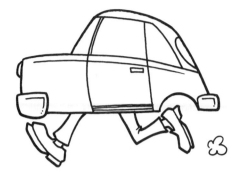

Chapter 21

Working Out on the Road

In This Chapter

➤ Traveling is not an excuse for not working out

➤ Calisthenics can save you

➤ Conquering jet lag drag

➤ Exercising high or low

➤ Being ready for any weather

Between work and play, many of us spend a few weeks on the road. For most, traveling is usually welcome, even if it often does throw you off your workout routine. People who travel a lot often say they can't work out, when in fact they choose not to. Taking a break is a good thing if you crave the rest; however, if you want to work out but don't because you're not sure of the options available to you, read on. There's plenty you can do, no matter where you are. As we see it, too may people become married to the exact routine that they've been doing week after week. Mixing up your routine is one of the best ways to improve your overall fitness; so actually breaking out of your fitness rut is an opportunity to do something new—not an excuse to do nothing. The issue isn't, "How the heck am I going to work out here?" but, "Let's see which workout I can pull from my bag of tricks."

Usually all that's required for you to keep working out on the road is an open mind with equal doses of planning and creativity. In this chapter, we'll guide you through strategies that will keep you sweating away from home, whether it's at a hotel gym, a nearby fitness center, park, or even in your room.

Seek and Ye Shall Find

Most hotels these days have either a modest facility where guests can work out or an affiliation with a health club that allow guests to train at a discounted rate. If you're lucky enough to stay at a hotel with decent facilities, you're in the chips. All you need to do is find the time to squeeze in a quick workout. (Or a long one if you have plenty of downtime.) However, if the hotel you're staying in doesn't have a gym or an arrangement with a gym, don't fret, there are still options available to you.

As we discussed earlier, if your health club is an International Health Racquet and Sportsclub Association (IHRSA) member, find out from their affiliation list if there is a gym near your hotel. During their vacation in San Francisco a few years ago, Deidre and Jonathan found three different health clubs in the IHRSA network and worked out at each of them during their week's stay. Each offered different machines and it was a good opportunity to try out a variety of equipment. (Although they did have to ask where the water fountain was each time.) If there is no convenient IHRSA facility, then you can always find the nearest gym and buy a day pass.

Not long ago, "World Pass for Fitness," an organization with travelers in mind, was created. This umbrella organization is basically a network of clubs throughout the country that must meet certain quality criteria to be accepted. The network accepts no more than one club per zip code. By paying a $79 fee (additional family members are $59), you're eligible to use any of the gyms within the national network. Before you crafty bargain hunters start thinking that you can use your local health club year-round for only $79, you should know that members are limited to three visits per week, six per month, and nine per year. In addition, you're not allowed to use a facility that's within 75 miles of your home. For more information about location and accommodations, you can check their Web site at www.worldpassforfitness.com.

With the IHRSA and/or the World Pass, you should be able to work out almost anywhere in the country. If you're outside of the country, you're still likely to find hotels with some gym facilities.

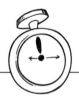

Short Cuts

A day pass can cost anywhere from $10 to $15. Ask at your home gym whether it is an IHRSA member. If it is, request a listing of gyms that are also in the network in the area that you plan to travel to.

Gym-less in Seattle

If you still can't find a gym near where you're staying, or if you think that working out in a new gym is intimidating or a waste of money, don't worry, we have something for you, too.

On a trip to Boston, Deidre went to the Women's Health Club, leaving Jonathan behind with nothing much to do. (He considered entering the women's-only establishment incognito but thankfully decided against it.) Instead of donning a wig and falsies, Jonathan went to a nearby park—a crude but very effective gym with clean air, plenty of room, and no lines. He did pull-ups on the monkey bars, push-ups, and crunches, and then went for a run. While he drew a few stares from some of the picnickers in the park, he enjoyed a good workout without dealing with any of the waiting or loud music that is the occupational hazards in many gyms.

Cals

Few gym owners and fitness trainers will tell you this, but calisthenics are an incredibly practical tool in your fitness arsenal. (If all people did was calisthenics, all gyms would be out of business.) Perhaps one of the reasons people don't do more of these time-efficient, extremely effective exercises is simple: They're difficult.

Deidre's dentist is friends with a 50-year-old fellow who routinely does around 1,000 push-ups a day. (That's 10 sets of 100; that's a lot!) At first he asked, "How the heck do you do that?" His reply was: "I started with as many as I could do [around 25] and just added one each day. Before I knew it, I was doing more and more." By the way, this guy had the upper body of a fit guy half his age.

Of course, the point is you don't need a fancy trainer or a spiffy gym with high-tech equipment to stay fit. Alex Lowe, who was once considered the greatest mountaineer in the world, never lifted weights, but he had an upper body that seemed chiseled from stone. His secret? He used to do 300 pull-ups a day.

A good idea is to work out a basic routine while at home so that when you are away, you can run through it without wasting time trying to figure out what you're going to do.

Here's a variety of exercises you can do while traveling.

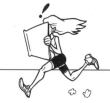

Info to Go

Herschel Walker, the great NFL running back and Olympic bobsledder, maintained his incredible physique with just push-ups and sit-ups. Of course, he did thousands a day.

Jumping Rope

Rope jumping is a tremendously challenging cardiovascular workout. Check back to Chapter 9, "The 15-Minute Cardio Workout," for some rope-jumping tips.

Push-Ups

When you're starting out, the key is doing them correctly. Perfect push-up form is described here:

1. Lie on the floor with legs together and hands on the floor pointing forward and just outside the shoulders.

2. Keep the back and legs straight.

3. Slowly push your body from the floor until your elbows are straight, then slowly return to the initial starting position. Keep your back straight. You can also change where you place your hands to emphasize different muscle groups. (Wide to emphasize the pecs, narrow for triceps.)

Pull-Ups and Chin-Ups

Pull-ups and chin-ups can be done on any horizontal object, but it's best to buy a chinning bar. Any exercise that relies on you pushing or pulling your body weight is going to be fairly challenging. Pull-ups and chin-ups can go a long way in building strength in several upper-body muscles. To do them properly …

1. Grab hold of the chinning bar with your hands several inches wider apart than shoulder width.

2. Keep your palms facing away from the body. Lift your feet off the floor and cross your legs at the ankles.

3. Pull your body up and touch the upper chest to the bar.

4. Pause briefly and return gradually to the initial starting position with your arms fully extended to get a good stretch.

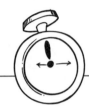

Short Cuts

The difference between the pull-up and the chin-up is the hand position. For pull-ups, palms face away from the body. For chin-ups, palms face toward the body. The underhand grip tends to stress the biceps muscles more, while the overhand emphasizes the muscles of the back more.

Resistance Bands

Resistance bands are basically giant rubber bands that provide resistance for exercises and can be used for variety of routines. Refer to Chapter 10, "The 15-Minute Strength-Training Workout," for some ideas on how to use bands.

Overcoming Jet Lag

Ask anyone who's flown a lot and he or she will have a good jet lag story for you. When Joe returned from China he was convinced he'd become a narcoleptic (someone who suffers from brief attacks of deep sleep). Ditto on his trip to South Africa. Of course, you can become a groggy mess just by taking the red-eye from New York to Los Angeles (or vise versa). Jet lag is a concern for all travelers who fly a lot.

For business travelers, however, it's much more difficult because you don't have the requisite time to recuperate, especially if you have to be sharp for the meeting that's often a few hours after you land. ("Nice effort, Johnson, but you seemed to be speaking in tongues.") While the dreaded jet lag is often unavoidable, this section will help you understand what causes it and how you can reduce it.

Just about everyone has a time of day where he or she feels more alert—your proverbial "morning" or "evening" person. These ups and downs throughout a 24-hour cycle is known as your *circadian rhythm*. Jet lag—or desynchronosis—interferes with the internal clock that we all have. Because you're zooming across a number of time zones in a matter of hours, the difference between where you are and where you were is flipped on its ear.

Jet lag can kick your behind in any number of negative ways:

➤ **Fatigue.** Often people lack concentration and motivation to do even basic things such as driving and reading. In addition, closing a multimillion-dollar business deal often becomes more difficult.

➤ **Disorientation, fuzziness.** A kissing cousin of fatigue, don't be surprised if you can't remember where you left your keys or where you parked your car.

➤ **Irrational, unreasonable behavior.** Blowing your stack over something inconsequential is bad form at any business meeting.

➤ **Broken sleep after arrival.** Remember your internal clock? Well, crossing time zones can cause you to wake up in the middle of the night and crave sleep during the day.

➤ **Dehydration.** This is a major problem on short hops, let alone major jaunts. Dehydration can cause headaches, dry skin, and nasal irritation as well as make you more susceptible to germs floating around the aircraft.

➤ **Swollen legs and feet.** Your limbs can swell while flying. In some cases this can prevent travelers from wearing their normal shoes for up to 24 hours after arrival.

➤ **Irregular bowel evacuation.** The World Health Organization (WHO) issued a report stating that jet lag is linked to problems with diarrhea caused by microbiological contamination of water or food. The report says this affects about 50 percent of long-distance travelers. "Factors such as travel fatigue, jet lag, a change

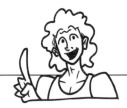

Workout Words

Circadian rhythm refers to an internal system in organisms that regulates behavior in a rhythmic manner, particularly events that occur at approximately 24-hour intervals, specifically the wake-sleep cycle.

in diet, a different climate, and a low level of immunity may aggravate the problem by reducing travelers' resistance and making them more susceptible to this type of infection or poisoning."

While you can't show your boss this section and tell him or her to give you a week of R and R before the "big" meeting, we can provide you with some techniques to reduce jet lag so that you arrive at your destination ready to perform at or near your best.

➤ **Preflight**. What you do before you step on the plane is one of the most important aspects of combating jet lag. First, don't hang out drinking the night before. Get plenty of exercise in the days before departure and try to avoid exposure to people with colds or the flu. If you have a cold, flying will probably make it worse. Delay the trip if you can; if you can't, make sure to get a good night's sleep the day before you head to the airport.

➤ **East or west?** There is data that holds that flying westward causes less jet lag than flying eastward. While this is an interesting tidbit, where you go on business is usually out of your control.

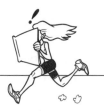

Info to Go

NASA estimates you need one day for every time zone crossed to regain normal rhythm and energy levels. For example, a five-hour time difference means you will require five days to get back to normal.

➤ **Day or night flight?** Many articles about time-zone traveling state that daytime flights cause less jet lag. While that may be so, we know many experienced travelers who find it best to leave at night, sleep for most of their flight, and arrive fresh at their destination.

➤ **Drinking fluids.** (And we don't mean vodka!) Many people assume that an alcoholic beverage will either calm their nerves and/or help them sleep. Good instinct, but it's generally a major mistake. Why? The dry air in the plane causes dehydration and drinking alcohol dehydrates you even more. Even drinking coffee, another diuretic, is usually a bad move. The best beverage to have while flying is good old water.

➤ **Sleeping aids.** Unless you're someone like Deidre, who can sleep at a construction site, you might need some assistance. Many people do well with a blindfold to block out the light and earplugs to quiet the noise. Since neck pain is a common complaint, an orthopedic neck rest can be the difference between tortured dozing and some solid Z's. Also removing your shoes and wearing slippers can up your comfort factor enormously.

➤ **Move as much as you can while on the plane.** This sounds goofy, but if you walk up and down the aisle, stand and stretch at least every two hours, it helps to reduce swelling in your legs and feet as well as the possibility of blood clots. Also, if there is a layover, get off and walk.

➤ **Seek light.** If it's daylight when you arrive at your destination, try and spend some time outdoors, since the sunlight will help to reset your internal clock. Again, try and avoid alcohol, caffeine, and rich foods. All of them can artificially affect your sleep patterns. Wake up in the morning at the appropriate local time, even if you don't have to. This will further help you adjust to the local time zone.

While we have no practical experience and can't endorse any of the following medicines we list below, there are a few supplements that are said to reduce the effects of jet lag. You should check with your physician before taking it.

➤ **No-Jet-Lag.** This is a homeopathic remedy in tablet form and is sold at international airports, pharmacies, and travel stores all over the world.

➤ **Melatonin.** Melatonin is a hormone secreted by the pineal gland, which is a pea-sized structure located in the center of the brain. Melatonin is produced during the night to assist our bodies in regulating our sleep-wake cycles. There is evidence to suggest that melatonin supplementation can help induce sleep and adjust you to the new time zone.

➤ **Sleeping pills are a bad idea.** Even for use as a sleep aid during your normal routine. They provide you with an altered state of sleep, overriding normal sleep patterns and leaving you feeling groggy upon waking. On a plane, the ramifications can be dangerous since sleeping pills put you in a near-comatose state. (There is very little natural movement, and movement is extremely important on a long flight.) When blood doesn't circulate, it clots, leaving you susceptible to *phlebitis* and stroke (if the clot moves from your leg to your brain). Also, be careful because some sleeping pills are variations on antihistamines, which tend to further dehydrate you.

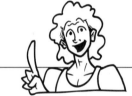

Workout Words

Phlebitis is the inflammation of a vein characterized by pain and tenderness along the course of the vein, discoloration of skin, inflammation and acute swelling below the obstruction, rapid pulse, mild elevation of temperature, and pain in the joints.

High Altitude

When John Krakauer's book *Into Thin Air* hit the best-seller list it was common cocktail conversation to talk about the lethal effects of high altitude. However, you don't have to head above 20,000 feet to learn a lot about thin air. Anyone who lives at sea level and rents a ski house in the Rockies will quite quickly start huffing and puffing while doing even routine tasks such as walking up a flight of stairs.

The key word here is *time,* since the body requires about eight days to fully acclimate to altitudes of 6,000 feet or more. During this time of acclimation, the body is making more red blood cells to adjust to the thinner air and decreased oxygen level. When Joe went to Quito, Ecuador, a bustling city surrounded by volcanoes at over 8,000 feet, he initially felt like he had a mild hangover he couldn't shake. After a few days, he felt simply drunk. Actually, in a day he felt fine. Only when he ventured above 13,000 feet did he really feel punk. For those of you who have never experienced life on a higher plane, we've noted the possible problems that can develop:

➤ Headaches.

➤ Agitation.

➤ Nausea and/or vomiting.

➤ General fatigue and ill feeling.

➤ Loss of appetite.

➤ Sleeplessness.

While people who are fit tend to suffer less from the effects of high altitude, often marathon runners suffer, and a duffer adapts without much of a problem. The bottom line is that you shouldn't begin a new exercise program when traveling someplace that's above a mile high. If you enjoy walking and hiking, go slow, drink plenty of water, and be mindful of the following distress symptoms during exercise:

➤ Shortness of breath.

➤ Rapid breathing.

➤ Increased heart rate.

➤ Fatigue with little effort.

If you experience any of the above, slow your pace, take time to rest, and continue drinking plenty of fluids. (Be careful of alcohol and caffeine.) If the symptoms don't dissipate, go to a lower altitude if possible.

Working Out in Bad Weather

Unless you live in San Diego or Tahiti, exercising in lousy weather is something that we all have to contend with—at home and on the road. Typically it's a matter of personal preference; some people don't mind running or walking in inclement weather, some tolerate it, others hate it and complain constantly. (Usually the rule of thumb is, when the weather gets tough, the tough head indoors to the gym.)

While Jonathan doesn't flinch when he has to do a bike race in rain, cold, or wind, he'll never train outside in the stuff, opting instead to ride on rollers indoors. Deidre, on the other hand, doesn't like to go outside if the thermometer dips below 72° or above 78°. This winter, the fair-weather couple was in a cab driving to the airport to fly to South Beach to escape the cold. It had snowed a couple of days earlier, and as they rolled through the slushy, miserable muck it began to rain. Moments later, they spotted a lone female runner running resolutely through all of that mess. While they admired her gumption, they were ecstatic they weren't where she was.

While this isn't a problem for most workout folks, it is a bugaboo for dedicated runners and walkers who really crave that endorphin fix that aerobic exercise provides. At home, it's less of a concern since you have access to appropriate clothing. When you travel, however, you rarely have the luxury of packing foul-weather rain gear. If you really want to be prepared, you can check to see what the weather will be during the days you will be away. That way if rain is predicted, you can pack accordingly. If you're on the road during the winter (Chicago, anyone?), think layers (see Chapter 23, "The Workout Wardrobe"). It's often a good idea to bring two pairs of sneakers, since wet sneakers may take more than a day to dry.

The Least You Need to Know

➤ You can usually find a gym with a reasonable daily fee.

➤ Calisthenics are efficient, effective, and available whenever you need them.

➤ Know how to stay fresh and ready for your business meeting when traveling across time zones.

➤ If you are traveling to a high-altitude region, you need to understand its effects on the body before attempting vigorous activity.

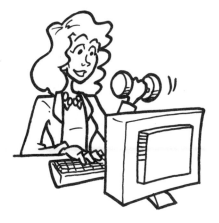

Chapter 22

Five-Minute Workouts at the Office

In This Chapter

➤ Avoiding carpal tunnel syndrome

➤ Choosing the right seat: the highs and lows

➤ Work fitness for everyone

➤ Clench your teeth to relax your mind

In theory, technology is supposed to help us work less (or at least more efficiently), but in the last few years it seems as if people sleep less and work more. Portable computers, cell phones, and the Internet allow us diligent office types to work even when we're on vacation. From a physiology point of view, this is a recipe for disaster. Headaches, backaches, and neck pain are frequently the by-products of this all-work and no-play lifestyle. As the saying goes, "Too much work and no play makes Johnny a physical wreck." Obviously, there must be a better way.

Odds are, if you have one of these all-consuming jobs that leaves you little time to butter your bagel in the morning, you're not going to be able to sit your boss down and tell him that the rigors of your job is hurting your 10K time. (First, he probably won't have enough time to hear you out and second, it's not his problem, it's yours.)

In this chapter we outline a handful of easy-to-do routines that you can do in five minutes (or less) throughout your workday. No, we won't have you doing sit-ups under your desk—though we're all for it. Rather, the intent here is to help relax your body as well as provide stress relief for your mind. Some are all-purpose exercise to help keep you in shape; others are specifically designed to counteract all of those sedentary hours at the desk.

Carpal Tunnel Syndrome

It's called *carpal tunnel syndrome,* or *CTS* (a form of *repetitive stress injury*) and it's often associated with carpenters or other manual laborers who perform repetitive skills with their hands. However, CTS is also a common problem for people who spend most of their time on a desktop or laptop computer. Twenty-seven percent of employee lost time is due to repetitive stress and carpal tunnel syndrome. On average, 40 workdays are used for sick time or rehabilitation of these injuries.

How can you decrease the likelihood of getting CTS or RSI? Short of winning the lottery or quitting your job to become a talk show host, there are a few strategies to keep in mind. First, make sure your desk is properly fit to your body. The second is to make sure you take frequent breaks during your busy day to stretch.

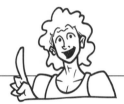

Workout Words

Carpal tunnel syndrome (CTS) is compression on the median nerve at the wrist. In your wrist there is a tunnel through which the median nerve and nine tendons pass. The median nerve supplies sensation to the thumb, index finger, middle finger, and half of the ring finger. Pain and/or numbness or tingling is felt in these digits when the wrist is bent at an acute angle.

While CTS centers around the wrist and the median nerve, **repetitive stress injuries (RSI)** can affect the neck, shoulders, upper back, and forearms, basically any body part that is repeating the same movement over the course of several hours. Sufferers feel pain from weakness and fatigue and are prone to tendinitis.

Try the following stretches.

The forearm and fingers stretch:

1. Rest your left forearm on the edge of your desk or chair.
2. Grasp the fingers of your left hand and gently bend back your wrist for 20 seconds.
3. Repeat with the other hand.

Hand press:

1. Gently press your hand against your desk with your palms down.

2. Stretch out your fingers and wrist for 20 seconds.

3. Repeat with the other hand.

Loose fist press:

1. Make a loose fist with your right hand.

2. Press it against the palm of your left hand, making sure to keep your right wrist straight. Hold each press for five seconds in the following positions:

   ➤ Palms down.

   ➤ Thumb up.

3. Repeat with the other hand.

Finger fan:

1. Tightly clench both of your hands, relax your fingers, and fan them out 10 times.

As always, staying limber before a problem occurs is the best way to avoid CTS or RSI. If you feel any tightness or discomfort in your hands or wrists, the best way to avoid further problems is to take frequent breaks. And it's really important to make sure that your desk, computer, chair, and phone are user friendly. Ergonomically designed keyboards make a big difference; ditto for chairs, and any other equipment you use routinely during your day.

Perfect Posture

"Sit up straight" may have been something your mom or teacher barked at you as a child. As annoying as it may have been, there was good reason for their reminders, especially if you spend much of your day at a desk working at a computer. This is extremely easy to do when talking about a desktop since one component can be positioned independently of the other. For example, a laptop is a self-contained unit. If the desk where you are working is too high or too low there is little you can do to make a better in relation to your total posture. A desktop, on the other hand, can be set up so that the keyboard is the appropriate height for your wrists and the monitor is the appropriate height for your head.

Take a Seat

The classic mistake that people make regarding chairs is thinking that bigger is better. In fact, the bigger the chair, the more likely it is that you will slouch in that cushy chair as if you're getting ready to munch on a bowl of popcorn and watch a movie on your computer.

Clearly, proper posture is crucial, but a proper-fitting chair is essential as well. Just as you wouldn't put a lanky six-foot-two guy on a bicycle designed for someone a foot shorter, the same rules apply in your regular old work chair. (Except that you spend far more time sitting at your desk than you do on your bicycle.)

Of course, as any good desk salesman could tell you, chairs don't exist in a vacuum. Where there is a chair there is more than likely a desk with a computer sitting on it. If your chair is too high, this increases flexion of your wrists as you type—making you a prime candidate for CTS. And if your chair is too low, the same thing happens for the opposite reason. And in either case, an improperly fitted chair changes the way you look at your computer monitor, which can affect your neck as well.

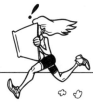

Info to Go

One of the things that Deidre found out early on when treating patients for neck and back pain was that the chairs they use at the office are the wrong height. Too small a chair means more slouching because their knees are bent higher than they should be, causing more flexion in their back. This means people have to crane their neck upward and before you can say "ergonomically correct," you've got people with neck pain, middle-back strain, and lower-back stiffness. Conversely, a chair that's too big forces you to sit on the edge without back support, which generally translates to discomfort and even pain.

What to Look For in a Chair

Height

Each chair should be adjustable to accommodate your size and desk height.

Arm Rests

Armrests should also be adjustable so that your elbows, when resting on the armrests, bend at a 90° angle.

Back Support

Look for a chair that has a slightly raised area that rests against your lumbar spine when you sit back in the chair. This slightly raised area will keep you in an erect-sitting posture.

Proper Workstation Posture

While most people understand how to sit properly when they're working, it's incredible how often we fall into bad habits. The key is to remind yourself to do the do's and avoid the don'ts. Once you ingrain the do's into your body memory, you're in the chips. To keep from lapsing into bad habits, it's a good idea to tape a list of the do's by your computer.

Posture Do's and Don'ts

Do's

Sit all the way back in your chair, not at the edge of your seat, which makes you prone to slumping.

Keep your neck and back facing forward, not up, down, or sideways.

Keep your knees slightly lower than your hips, which encourages erect sitting posture.

Keep your elbows bent at a 90° angle when using the keyboard.

Keep your wrists in a neutral position when using the keyboard. If your wrists are angled up when using the keyboard, purchase an ergonomic wrist pad to attach to the front of the keyboard.

Keep your entire foot on the floor or footrest.

Don'ts

Cross your legs.

Sit on the edge of the chair.

Shift weight to one side.

Sit on one leg.

Put your feet up on the desk.

Setting Up an Ergonomically Efficient Workstation

In addition to how the mouse, keyboard, and monitor should be set up, there are a couple of other important placements that you should be aware of.

➤ **Screen:** Your screen should be able to tilt up and down as well as swivel from side to side.

➤ **Viewing distance:** The best distance to be from the screen when working on your computer is between 18 and 24 inches. You should also purchase an antiglare screen that fits on to your computer screen.

➤ **Telephone:** Talk to anyone who uses the phone all day—from stockbrokers to taxi dispatchers—and odds are they're using a hands-free head set that allows you to maintain proper head positioning while talking on the phone and working at your computer. Go without it for any length of time and your head is likely to be permanently tipped to one side.

Setting up your workstation protects the well-being of your neck, back, shoulders, and wrists.

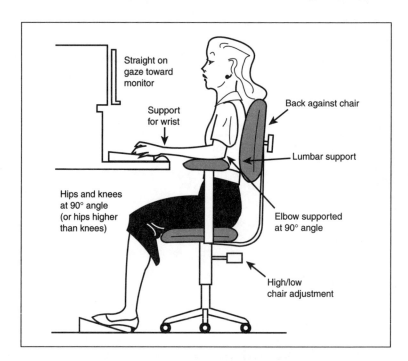

Combating Neck, Back, and Shoulder Pain

Let's assume that your workstation is as ergonomically effective as Lance Armstrong's time-trial bicycle, but you're still stiff and achy halfway through you day. Now what do you do?

No matter how well your desk is set up, you were not meant to remain in a static position for hours on end. Sleep or sit too long and you usually feel stiff as a board. To keep blood flowing through your muscles and fluid through your joints it's important to move at regular intervals. This means you should get up every 20 to 30 minutes and move, move, move!

Stretching at Your Desk

Working can literally be a pain in the neck (not to mention a headache). That's because poor posture and stress often lead to the shortening of your trapezius, levator scapula, and cervical spinal extensor muscles. For relief, try the following stretches.

Trapezius stretch:

1. Sit up straight in your chair.
2. Place your right hand on the left side of your head.
3. Gently pull your head toward your right shoulder until you feel a slight stretch.
4. Hold for 20 to 30 seconds.
5. Repeat on the other side.

Be careful not to hunch your shoulders as you perform this stretch.

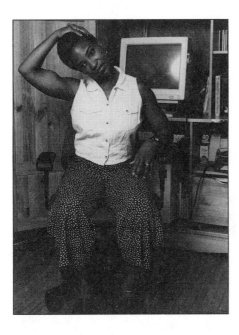

You'll feel this stretch through the side of your neck.

Levator scapula stretch:

1. Sit up straight in your chair.
2. Look down toward your right hip.
3. Place your right hand on your head and gently pull your head toward your right hip.
4. Hold for 20 to 30 seconds.
5. Repeat on the other side.

This stretch is great for your neck and shoulders after hours of staring at a computer monitor.

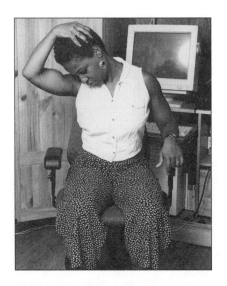

The chin tuck:

1. Sit up straight in your chair.

2. Imagine a string attached to the top of your head. Now imagine someone pulling up on the string and tuck your chin back and in as your neck lengthens.

3. Repeat 10 times.

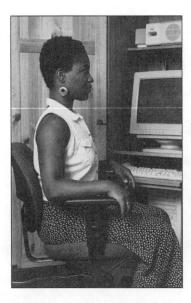

Begin the chin tuck with your head in a neutral position.

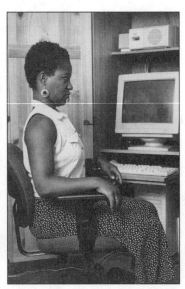

You'll know you've done the chin tuck properly if you have a double chin when you do it.

The pectoral (chest) muscles are often shortened because of poor posture. A good way to lengthen those muscles is to do this pectoral stretch. Refer to Chapter 7, "Start with Stretching," for the proper pectoral stretch. Sorry, but this stretch requires you to get up out of your chair.

Back extension:

1. Stand up and put your hands on your hips.

2. Lean backward as far as you can comfortably.

3. Hold for 20 to 30 seconds.

4. Keep your head in neutral, don't look backward (you can get dizzy and throw your balance off).

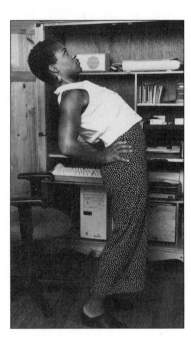

The back extension feels great after you've been in a chair for hours.

Side stretch:

1. Stand up and put your left hand on your hip.

2. Lean over toward your left side as far as you can comfortably.

3. Bring your right arm up and reach toward your left side.

4. Hold for 20 to 30 seconds.

5. Repeat on the other side.

269

This is another effective stretch when you've been sitting all day.

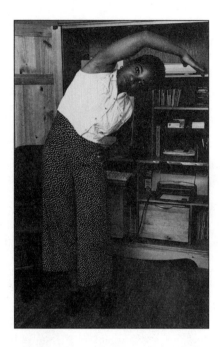

Strengthening at Your Desk

Just as there are muscles that become shortened and tight when you're sitting at your desk, there are other muscles that become too stretched. In particular, the scapula (shoulder blade) muscles, rhomboids, and middle trapezius are often sites of muscle spasm and fatigue because of poor posture. To combat this, it's best to do strengthening work.

Scapula retraction:

1. Sit straight in your chair.
2. Bring your arms to your side and bend your elbows to 90°.
3. Squeeze your shoulder blades together, holding for five seconds.
4. Repeat 10 to 15 times.

Your forearm muscles that are attached to your elbow make your wrists move. If these muscles are not strong they may fatigue and become prone to tendinitis. To keep your forearm muscles in good functioning shape, do the following:

Forearm extension:

1. Sit erect in a chair with armrests.
2. Place your arms on the chair, with your hands facing palms down over the edge of the armrest.

3. Making a loose fist, bring your wrists slowly up then slowly down.

4. Repeat 10 to 15 times.

Forearm flexion:

1. Sit erect in a chair with armrests.

2. Place your arms on the chair, with your hands facing palms up over the edge of the armrest.

3. Making a loose fist, bring your wrists slowly up then slowly down.

4. Repeat 10 to 15 times.

Although you may not think so, sitting on your rump all day can be tough on your lower body. Keep the blood flowing in your butt and legs by doing the following:

Gluteus squeezes:

1. While sitting in your chair, squeeze your buttocks together.

2. Hold each squeeze for five seconds and release.

3. Repeat 10 to 15 times.

Quadriceps/hamstring squeezes:

1. While sitting in your chair, tighten your hamstring and quadriceps muscles.

2. Hold each squeeze for five seconds and release.

3. Repeat 10 to 15 times.

Calf raises:

1. Stand behind your chair.

2. Raise up on your toes.

3. Slowly lower yourself.

4. Repeat 20 times.

These exercises will help you become aware of tense muscles and get a little blood flowing to the problem areas.

Stair Workouts

Think of the stairs in your office building as a built-in piece of gym equipment. If you're unable to do any aerobic exercising during the day (or week), they're always there. If you're working out regularly, it's a great way to augment your routine. In fact, football players, track and field athletes, rowers, and basketball players all run stairs to build leg and cardiovascular strength. If stairs are good enough for athletes

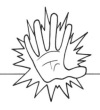

Stop Short

When you begin walking up stairs, don't attack them like an NFL running back. Try this instead. If your office is on the fifth floor, walk up instead of taking the elevator. Don't hustle; Just walk up at a moderate pace so that you can carry on a conversation. If you can, take the stairs two at a time.

to train on, they're certainly good enough for the rest of us. While huffing up flights of stairs isn't a ball of laughs, it's a very efficient and effective exercise.

While climbing stairs will get you fitter, the exercise will increase your circulation and help make you more alert. Also, when you've been focused on one thing for an extended period, doing something physical is a good way to give your brain a break. Often people find that when they step away from a particular problem and get out and walk around, the solution pops into their head.

During the day, especially if you've been stuck on a problem, saunter over the staircase and walk up two or three flights of stairs. Control your breathing—no panting or gasping—and try not to think about your work. Continue to do this every day, adding a full flight each day until you are able to climb for 10 continuous minutes.

Calisthenics Are Convenient

The best thing about calisthenics is that you can use them wherever you are, at home, in the hotel, in the office. Now, we don't expect you to drop down and give 20 in the boardroom or beside the water cooler, but if you pick your spots (especially if you have an office with a door), you'll be able to do a few of the exercises we list below.

Performing Push-Ups

We all know how standard push-ups are performed: nose to the floor, hands shoulder-width apart, toes touching, body just inches off the ground. Down, up, down, until you finish your set. Office decorum, however, demands something a touch subtler:

Modified push-ups:

1. Stand approximately three feet away from a wall.
2. Place your hands against the wall just outside of your chest at chest level.
3. Tighten your abdominals.
4. Slowly lower your chest to the wall.
5. Hold this position for five seconds, then slowly return to your starting position.
6. Don't allow your abdominals to sag toward the wall.
7. Repeat 15 times.

Chair dips:

1. Position yourself on the edge of a nonrolling chair.
2. Stretch your feet out in front of you as you slide yourself off the chair so only your hands remain on the chair's edge.
3. Slowly lower your buttocks toward the floor.
4. Slowly return to your starting position.
5. Repeat 15 times.

Contract/Relax Technique

Tension is as common in the workplace as donuts and coffee. Often it's so pervasive we don't even know that we're tense until we notice that our teeth are clenched and our shoulders are up around our ears. A good technique that Deidre has many of her patients do is "contract/relax." It's easy to do and can be done in the office, waiting on the deli line, or in a cab. Use this in conjunction with deep breathing to relax yourself when you feel those shoulders tensing.

1. Squeeze your eyes shut, hold for five seconds, then relax.
2. Clench your teeth, hold for five seconds, then relax.
3. Hunch your shoulders up toward your ears, hold, then relax.
4. Squeeze your shoulder blades together, hold, then relax.
5. Squeeze your fingers together into a fist, hold, then relax.
6. Squeeze your buttocks together, hold, then relax.
7. Tighten your thigh muscles, hold, then relax.
8. Curl your toes together, hold, then relax.
9. Tighten everything, hold as you count to five, then relax.

When you realize what it feels like when you're tense, you can catch yourself and consciously relax. It's a simple technique that will go a long way toward combating muscle spasms and chronic fatigue.

The Least You Need to Know

➤ An ergonomically correct workstation is key to a healthy work environment.

➤ Walk up the stairs to rev up your metabolism and brainpower.

➤ Modifications to the standard calisthenics routine can make them handy to do anywhere.

➤ Contract/relax techniques can give you the power to destress anytime.

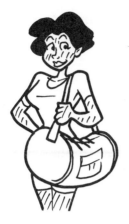

Chapter 23

The Workout Wardrobe

In This Chapter

➤ Materials to keep cool and dry

➤ Layering for comfort

➤ Choosing the right footwear

➤ Equipment for home or the road

Tennis star Andre Agassi once said: "Image is everything." (Of course, he was paid big bucks to say that, so who knows if he actually believed it.) But to anyone who works out regularly, the more important credo is "comfort and function is everything." Sure you want to look good, but if your workout wear doesn't fit well, doesn't dry quickly or breathe effectively, well, as we say in Brooklyn, you're blank out of luck. Considering that your authors spend as much (or more) time in workout clothes than most businesspeople do a suit, this is a subject near and dear to us.

In this chapter, we'll give you a basic overview of the different kinds of garments you can use depending on the activity you're doing and when you're doing it. We'll also give you some insights about one of our favorite subjects: footwear. Finally, we'll give you the skinny on portable exercise equipment that you can use (unobtrusively) at home, as well as stuff to carry with you when you're on the road.

Threads

If you live in San Diego and split your workout time between the gym with an occasional jog at the beach, then you can probably skip this section. However, if it rains more than eight times a year where you reside, where the temperature can swing 15°

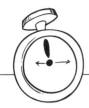

Short Cuts

Good workout clothing can sometimes be a bit pricey, but it's a good idea to invest in good quality. Pay special attention to any items that will be against your skin, as lower-end items can often cause skin irritation from exposed seams.

to 20° in a day, read on, since knowing what to wear and what contingencies to make can mean the difference between comfort and misery.

At the 1999 five-mile Turkey Trot in Prospect Park, New York, on a chilly Thanksgiving morning, Jonathan and Deidre ran with a friend who decided to run in her sweatpants and sweatshirt. Clad in Patagonia lyrax long-sleeve tops and Lycra shorts, Jonathan and Deidre were far from comfortable in the driving rain, but they were also far from chilled, since the skintight material breathes and helps retain body heat. Contrast that with their friend in the sweats. Not only did she weigh 20 pounds more at the end of the race, but she also was as cold as a wet rag stuck in the refrigerator.

While this tops the list of what *not* to wear, it does take a bit of experimentation to see what garments work under what conditions. The other important thing is learning the layering game (more on that later).

Form Meets Content

Let's look at some of the basic garments you should have in your workout wardrobe.

Running Shorts

When they start running, many people assume they can wear anything to pound the pavement—an old pair of cutoff jeans, Bermuda shorts, you name it. While there's no arguing that you can run in just about anything, it's not until they try on a comfortable pair of running shorts that they say, "Wow, this makes running much easier." Light, quick drying, and available in a variety of lengths, running shorts come with a built-in undergarment. Check any good running store or running shoe catalogue and you'll see how many companies make these nifty shorts. In our opinion, Desoto Sport makes some of the best. In addition, running shorts can double for any gym activity from lifting to the StairMaster.

Cycling Shorts

Cycling shorts are the Jekyll and Hyde of fitness garments. Ride without them and they're sorely missed; wear them to walk around town in and you can't wait to change into something more comfortable. Unlike regular shorts that would billow as you ride, these form-fitting Lycra shorts with the padded seat protect your thighs from chaffing as you pedal over hill and dale. For precisely that same reason, they can be irritating if you were to wear them on a hike or on the tennis court. One word of caution: The seams on the padding can be uncomfortable, so try them on before you buy. Jonathan, who rides roughly 5,000 miles a year, favors shorts by Pearl Izumi.

For Women Only: Sports Bras

Sports bras are an invaluable part of a woman's fitness wardrobe, especially for full-figured women. There are three things to remember when choosing a sports bra: proper fit, comfort, and structure.

➤ **Fit.** When shopping for a sports bra, always try it on before you buy it. Once you try it on, clap your hands overhead; if the plastic band moves up your chest, it's too tight. You don't want to worry about flashing your gym mates while you're exercising.

➤ **Comfort.** Remember, be practical. If it looks good but isn't comfortable, it isn't worth it.

➤ **Structure.** There are two types of sports bras to choose from: compression and encapsulation. Compression bras press the breasts against the chest in a single mass and work best for small to medium-sized breasts. The encapsulation style is akin to the brassiere; they hold each breast separately. This works best for full-figured women.

Singlets

Singlets are lightweight, sleeveless or short-sleeved tops typically used by runners and triathletes and cyclists (when it's quite warm). If it's hot and you want to wear something, a quick-drying singlet is the way to go. You can also wear it as a second layer over a heavier closer-to-skin garment to add a bit of insulation. This is often a good move when you're out for a bike ride.

Socks

Joe has 987 socks but only possesses four or five matching pairs in good condition that he pulls out for races and other important occasions. That's because a good pair of lightweight comfortable socks offers cushioning when you run, helps keep your feet dry, prevents blisters, and just plain feels good. Of course, in the winter when you hit the slopes you'll need a thicker pair (or two) but the same principles apply. Jonathan swears by Thorlo; Joe is fond of any sport socks that match and fit.

Material Matters

The right material can make the difference between you finishing your workout relatively comfortable or a sweaty, soggy mess. The right high-tech fabrics are an exerciser's best friend.

Lycra/Spandex

These fabrics were developed in the 1950s to take the place of rubber materials that were used in undergarments such as brassieres and girdles. Lycra and Spandex are blended with natural and man-made fibers including cotton, wool, silk, and linen and they are much lighter than their rubber thread predecessors. In addition, they don't break down with exposure to body oils, perspiration, lotions, or detergents. The form-fitting nature of Lycra and Spandex is not just for the sake of aesthetics. The tight but stretchy nature helps prevent rubbing and chafing. Lycra and Spandex are well known for their ability to stretch despite the fact that they're skintight. They're comfortable, help keep you dry, and come in roughly 10 million colors.

Cotton

If you're like Jonathan or Joe, guys who've done countless races, you have anywhere from 50 to 300 T-shirts piled in your closet. While these are great mementos that you can wear when you're lifting weights in the gym, cotton is the absolute worst fabric to wear when you're getting sweaty outdoors. (In fact, it's fairly lousy indoors as well, but at least you won't freeze.) That's because cotton retains sweat and prevents evaporation. As a result, you feel cold and clammy; however, because your sweat evaporates so slowly your body has to work harder to keep you cool.

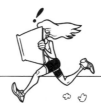

Info to Go

It might please you to know that even the so-called "experts" make mistakes. While training for the 1999 New York City Marathon, Deidre went for a run in Brooklyn's Prospect Park during the late fall, wearing a jog bra under a cotton shirt. For the first 20 minutes she was fine on this cool afternoon; however, once she hit her stride the wind picked up and her sweaty shirt left her colder by the minute. By the time she got home, her teeth were chattering. Had she worn a Thermax top layer over her jog bra, she would have been much warmer and drier. The moral of the story is not to wear the commemorative race T-shirt for the race.

CoolMax

Unlike cotton, CoolMax is a polyester fabric that pulls sweat away from the body to the outer layer. This allows for the moisture to evaporate, keeping you cool and dry.

The difference you feel when you wear CoolMax versus cotton is enormous. According to Dupont, the manufacturer of CoolMax, garments made with CoolMax dried almost completely in 30 minutes—roughly twice as fast as cotton. Whether you're running a marathon or paddling a kayak, this ultralight garment is so efficient at wicking away moisture it's almost as if you're wearing nothing at all. Jonathan often wears a sleeveless CoolMax shirt under his cycling uniform, and finds that it actually feels cooler than without the additional layer. CoolMax is also available with long sleeves, which is a great base layer for cooler weather.

One product that we especially like are shorts and tights called "Lycra Power," available through a company called Sweat It Out. Made of a mix of 30 percent Lycra and 70 percent CoolMax, the material provides a lot of stretch and compression and may even help prevent hamstring injuries by preventing muscle vibration. (Think of the layer a lot of NBA players wear under their baggy shorts.) More studies are needed to confirm these preliminary results, but the ever-skeptical Jonathan swears by them and wears them under his running shorts all the time.

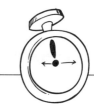

Short Cuts

One common complaint about CoolMax is that even after you wash it several times it smells like an old sock. We've had good results with after-wash deodorant sprays such as Febreze.

Lively in Layers

When you look at what outdoorsmen wore to brave the elements back in the "good old days"—animal skins, anyone?—and contrast that to the space-age technology available today, well, the good old days were better. Gore-Tex, CoolMax, Lycra, spandex, and a variety of other materials are the key decision an outdoor athlete has to make. And nowadays the best way to handle the conditions you experience when you're working out outside is to combine these garments.

Welcome to the refined art of layering. Layering clothing is important when you head into cold or inclement conditions. Whether you're running, cycling, kayaking, in-line skating, or just going out on a hike, how you layer your workout clothes is extremely important. Too little and you're freezing; too much and you're hot and cranky. Here's what you need to know.

Base Layer

The base layer is right next to your skin. The fabric you choose should draw sweat away from your skin to the outer layer to prevent you from feeling sweaty and hot in the summer or clammy and cold in the winter.

➤ Cold-weather choices: polypropylene (Capilene, Thermion, Thermax, Thermastat).

➤ Warm-weather choices: CoolMax, Supplex, or polyester microfiber.

Insulating Layer

For cooler weather you need a layer of warmth that you can easily remove if you get too hot. In really cold conditions, your choices for your upper and lower body are wool, fleece, pile, or down. For example, Jonathan likes to wear a fleece vest over his base layer of Thermax. Since it is sleeveless, chances are he won't overheat. If the weather is too cold for a vest, a long-sleeve pullover made of fleece would be appropriate. If you get too hot, you can remove it and tie it around your waist.

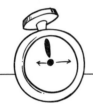

Short Cuts

Remember that in cold weather the rule of thumb is, the faster you move, the more layers you need. That's why you'll need to bundle up more for cycling or in-line skating than for running.

Outer Layer

The outermost layer protects you from the elements— usually wind, rain, or cold. If it's raining, you'll need a windproof/water-resistant jacket that "breathes." Gore-Tex and Ultrex are best.

It's important to note when it's cold outside that you actually want to be cool (not cold) when you start, since once you start working out you're going to heat up fast. If you're still cold after 10 to 15 minutes then you need to put on another layer. Also note that you'll stay warmer if your upper body is better insulated than bundling up your lower body and going light on top. A good pair of light gloves and a Lycra cap can help you maintain body heat.

Dress Code

Now that we've given you the rundown on what layer goes where, here are some tips as to when and where you can wear them.

At Home

In our own home, anything goes, including your purple polka-dotted pajamas, but if you plan to ride a stationary bike indoors we recommend cycling shorts. If you're on a treadmill, we recommend running shorts and a jog bra for women, running shorts and a singlet for men.

At the Gym

Here are some recommendations for clothing that will keep you comfortable while you work out at the gym.

➤ **Running:** Running shorts and sports bra and/or singlet is fine for the treadmill.

➤ **Spin class:** Cycling shorts and a sports bra and/or singlet.

➤ **Strength training:** If you're not going to be sweating bullets, any comfortable-fitting T-shirt should do the trick. Try and color coordinate with your shoes, socks, and wristbands.

➤ **Step class/aerobics:** Running shorts or midthigh shorts and a sports bra and/or singlet.

➤ **Yoga:** Loose-fitting clothing is best so you can stretch easily. Sweatpants, or cotton drawstring pants with a sports bra and/or singlet or comfortable T-shirt.

On the Road

When you travel you want to make sure that you're prepared for a variety of conditions. We sometimes get into trouble when we pack the gear that we need at home only to find that it's 15° cooler when we get off the plane. Picture the worst conditions you can expect in the place you're going and pack accordingly. You can be prepared for working out by bringing minimal gear.

➤ Running shorts.

➤ Sports bra.

➤ Lycra running pants.

➤ Singlet.

➤ Cap. (A baseball cap can keep your head warm and the sun out of your eyes.)

➤ Socks.

➤ Sneakers.

➤ Gore-Tex wind/rain proof jacket.

The above are all handy because they are lightweight, take up minimal space in your suitcase, and are easy to wash in the bathroom sink and drip-dry overnight.

Shoes

Years ago there were three types of sneakers: Pro Keds, Converse, and skips. If you aspired to be among the cool crowd, you wore either Keds or Cons. If you were in the egghead crowd (or too cool to care) you wore skips.

Nowadays, you name it and there is a sneaker for it: Even in the running shoe world there are umpteen types of shoes for training, racing, trail running, and more. There are so many types of athletic shoes available that even Imelda Marcos would be challenged to own them all. While there's obviously a big difference between rigid cycling shoes and wrestling shoes, for the general workout fan, any comfortable running or cross-training shoe should be fine.

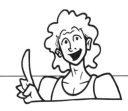

Workout Words

To **pronate** is to bear most of your weight on the inner portion of your foot. You can often tell by looking at the wear pattern on the sole of your shoes whether you pronate or **supinate** (to bear weight on the outer portion of your foot as you walk).

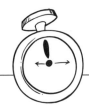

Short Cuts

A great way to tell whether you are a pronator, supinator, or average: Step out of the bathtub onto a bare floor. Look at the type of footprint you leave:

➤ If you see a clearly defined print of your heel, the balls of your toes, but a very slim outline of the outer portion of your foot you're a supinator.

➤ If you see your entire foot, you're a pronator.

➤ If you see most of foot except for the inner portion, you have a "normal" foot.

Fitting Your Foot

The type of sneaker that you choose obviously depends on the type of activity that you are doing and the type of foot that you have. People often ask us what's a good sneaker, as if there's one magical shoe that will work for everyone. Obviously you need to factor in the activity that you'll be doing, but you also need to consider what you bring to the equation. Your size and the structure of your foot are very important. First let's talk about foot type.

These are the basic questions that you should be able to answer about your feet.

➤ Are you flat-footed? (No arch.)

➤ Are you a *pronator?* (Walk on the inner portion of your foot, like most flat-footers do.)

➤ Do have a high arch?

➤ Are you a *supinator?* (Walk on the outer portion of your foot, like most high-archers do.)

If you're not sure, go to a store known for its sneaker savvy. The salesperson will have you take off your shoes and stand. By observing your feet, he or she will be able to answer those questions and recommend a shoe that may be appropriate. Never, however, just take a shoe based on a recommendation without trying it on. The shoe may be appropriate for all pronators except for you. And follow the old edict, "If the shoe fits, wear it." If you're a woman who feels more comfortable wearing a men's shoe, wear it.

Match Your Shoe to What You Do

The right type of sneaker depends on your chosen activity. If you plan to weight train and/or take an aerobics class (whether it be step or traditional) a cross-training shoe is your best bet because it offers you good arch support as well as good medial (inner) and lateral (outer) support.

If you plan to run more than once or twice per week, then your decision will be based on how many miles you log and your foot type and weight. The heavier you are, the more shock absorption you need, to minimize the pounding. Men weighing 180 pounds or women weighing 150 pounds will sorely appreciate a more cushioned shoe.

Generally, if you're flat-footed or pronate you'll need a running shoe that has good, solid medial (inner) post support. If you have a high arch or supinate, you will need a sneaker that has more midsole cushioning and less medial support. If you plan on racing 5Ks and 10Ks, you can train in a more cushioned (read heavier) pair. On race day, whip out your racing flats and have at it. You'll feel as if you're running on air. Don't, however, make the mistake of running a marathon in racing flats unless you're really light on your feet—well, you know what we mean.

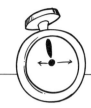

Short Cuts

When shopping for sneakers go in the afternoon when your feet are slightly swollen. Bring the socks you plan to wear with your sneakers to ensure a good fit.

Don't Resist Resistance Bands

Okay, you're on the road. You have limited time and can't be bothered with finding a gym. What to do? If you're like us, you might pull out your portable resistance bands. While it sounds like a subversive group of terrorists, the variety we're talking about are giant rubber bands that comprise a color-coded progressive resistance system. (Pink is the easiest and silver the hardest.) Refer to Chapter 10, "The 15-Minute Strength-Training Workout," on exercise routines with resistance bands.

Accessories are available to make the exercises more versatile, including exercise handles and door anchors. They enable you to work out with the bands with greater stability.

The best thing about these handy bands is their portability and relative efficiency when you're in a hotel or even in your office with some time to kill. We're not suggesting that you can get in great shape using them regularly, but their convenience is their biggest selling point.

Resistance Bands

Pros

Easy to pack.

Variable resistance.

Can be used for a variety of exercises.

Safe.

continues

Resistance Bands   (continued)

Cons

The resistance is not constant throughout the full range of motion (ROM).

While there are some good exercises to do for the smaller body parts like shoulders and arms, there are not many effective exercises to do for larger body parts like your glutes, quads, and hamstrings.

There is a limit to their shelf life—the more you use them, the more worn they get, leading to breaks in the band.

Another type of resistance that you may not have seen is the AquaBell Dumbbell Water System. As the name suggests, this is a portable water-inflatable system that is ideal for people who travel. They are easy to carry since they weigh only 24 ounces when collapsed; when filled with water, each dumbbell weighs up to 16 pounds.

AquaBells are great, portable dumbbells.

(Source: AquaBell)

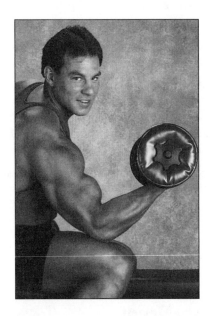

Ankle Weights Are Awesome

Ankle weights are perfect for use in the rehab setting because they can be easily adapted to be used with virtually any body part (dumbbells can be used most efficiently with only the upper extremity) whether it be shoulders, hips, or knees.

Just as there are many different dumbbells, ankle weights also come in more than one style (such as sand-filled ankle weights and lead-column ankle weights). Since lugging around an extra 10 or 20 pounds in your suitcase or briefcase may not be your idea of fun, AquaBell makes ankle weights as well.

They weigh only eight ounces when collapsed and inflate to eight pounds of resistance.

AquaBell Ankle Weight Water System

Pros

They're lightweight and take up little room in your suitcase.

They offer enough resistance to get a good workout.

They are made of tough, high-tech material that will last for years.

Unlike lead-column ankle weights, they won't set off alarms going through airport security.

Cons

There must be one, but we can't think of it right now.

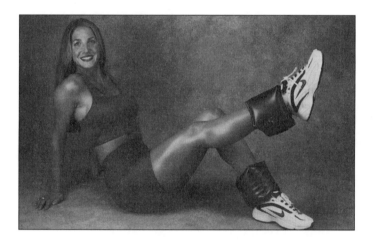

Just like the dumbbells, AquaBell ankle weights are easily packed away in a suitcase.

(Source: AquaBell)

The Least You Need to Know

➤ Understand the material that your workout clothing is made of and how it keeps you comfortable.

➤ There are clothes for running, riding, and lifting. Know what to wear and when.

➤ Sneakers are specialized so get the proper ones for your sport.

➤ You can get an effective and efficient workout with dumbbells, ankle weights, and resistance bands.

285

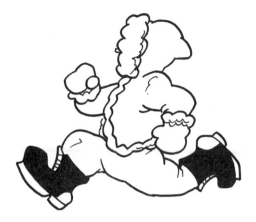

Chapter 24

Seasonal Workouts

In This Chapter

➤ How to handle working out in the heat

➤ Winter fun for everyone

➤ Avoiding the dangers of frostbite and heatstroke

➤ Safety first, use equipment, pay attention

It sounds ridiculously simple, but many people miss the obvious point when it comes to fitness, thinking of it as work rather than play. But staying physically fit should be about actively enjoying your surroundings, inside and out. While we're big "gym guys," much of the work we do in the gym is so that when we take our fitness outside we can enjoy it that much more. (Of course, being competitive lunatics ensures that we train hard so that we can race well.) The point remains: The more your fitness becomes play, the more it will remain a part of your life. If you want proof, just look at children. Running, jumping, and climbing in a playground is a joyous activity. They have no goals other than to have fun and their physicality is an expression of this inner joy. In fact, a great way to incorporate play into your fitness is to work out with pets and kids.

A commitment to fitness (to play) is a commitment no matter the weather. If you just work out indoors week after week you're bound to get bored. A good way to continue to be fit and to have fun is to get acquainted with sports that you can do in every season. It's a great way to cross-train and it keeps you motivated as well.

In this chapter we'll also give you a thumbnail sketch of what you can expect from a few of our favorite summer and winter sports.

Stay Warm in the Cold

When exercising in the winter, layers are the way to go. That's because you trap more and more air with each layer that you wear; the trapped air becomes warm, creating an effective layer of insulation. One of the most important articles of dressing for the cold is a hat, since approximately 30 percent to 40 percent of body heat is lost through the head. Wearing a wool hat goes a long way toward keeping you warm. Your workout attire depends on a number of factors: air temperature, wind velocity, and the kind of workout you hope to accomplish. When Jonathan ran the Mardi Gras Marathon in New Orleans, it was a balmy 38°F. Had he been training, he would have worn tights and a few layers with a windbreaker and hat. However, in an effort to balance his desire to feel loose and unencumbered with not wanting to freeze his behind off, he wore shorts and a sleeveless shirt with a baseball cap and gloves.

Another obvious benefit of layering is that when you get too warm you can shed clothes. This is where the type of material that you are wearing comes in. If you're wearing a natural fiber such as cotton, the moisture from your perspiration will make the clothing wet. When clothing gets wet it loses close to 90 percent of its insulating properties, causing more heat to be lost since water conducts heat much faster than air.

In the cold weather, blood is diverted from the extremities to the body's core to ensure that the major organs remain warm and continue to receive adequate oxygen for nutrition and metabolic waste removal. As a result, the temperature of the skin and the extremities can fall to dangerous levels. Early warning signs of cold injury are tingling and numbness in the fingers and toes and a burning sensation in the nose and ears. If these signs are ignored, overexposure can lead to tissue damage.

Choose your sport and route wisely depending on the type of day you have. If you are running, skiing, or skating into the wind, the wind-chill factor is related to how fast you are going. For example, running at 8 miles per hour into a 12-mile-per-hour headwind is the same as a 20-mile-per-hour wind speed. The same

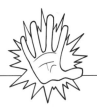

Stop Short

It is important to understand some of the ways that the body adjusts to exercising in both hot and cold weather. Knowing more about the warning signs of extreme weather illness such as frostbite, heat exhaustion, and heatstroke will help you dress appropriately and, more important, avoid them before things get serious.

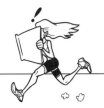

Info to Go

Cycling in the cold weather can be especially uncomfortable because of the wind chill factor even on calm days. That's because if you're moving at 20 miles per hour, you're creating your own wind. As a result, you'll need to throw on more layers to ride in 30° than if you were running in the same conditions.

holds true for running with a tail wind; an 8-mile-per-hour run with a 12-mile-per-hour wind at your back provides a relative wind speed of 4 miles per hour.

Winter Wonders

Durango, Colorado's Ned Overend has won one world championship to go along with six national mountain bike titles. While Durango is one of the great mountain biking towns in the country, in the winter the trails are buried by snow. Overend, who since retiring from the pro circuit has turned his attention to doing "extreme" triathlons, has a simple philosophy that boils down to don't fight the weather. In his view, winter is nature's way of making him take a break from riding. Instead of trying to ride in lousy weather he recommends participating in any other sport that you enjoy—soccer, basketball, swimming, snowshoeing, cross-country skiing, or martial arts. (He even likes Ping-Pong, which he says improves hand-to-eye coordination for mountain biking. However, unless you play for the Chinese Olympic team, Ping-Pong offers minimal fitness benefits.)

The key again is diversity and enjoyment. Now 44 and still fit enough to win the Xterra Triathlon Championship in Maui in 1998 and 1999 against pros half his age, Overend has been racing at an elite level for two decades. If it's good enough for him, it should be good enough for you. Here are some snapshots of a few of our favorite off-season activities.

Ice-Skating

In-line skating and ice-skating are similar enough to be considered kissing cousins. Both require good balance and specific skills including turning and stopping. (A valuable skill if you skate in the streets in the city.) If you're a cyclist, both sports offer excellent cross-training. If you opt for ice-skating indoors you won't have to dress as warm as you would for "blading" in the winter. However, you need to wear far fewer layers on in-line skates than

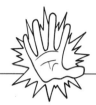

Stop Short

Asthmatics are prone to exercise-induced asthma attacks in either hot or cold weather; the risk is even higher during the cold. Prevent attacks in the cold by always wearing a scarf over your nose and mouth. And never exercise without your inhaler.

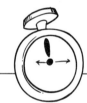

Short Cuts

When you're cycling or running in the winter, it's safer to head out into the wind because you can quickly determine if you're wearing enough clothing by facing the coldest weather first. More important, if you run out of energy on the run or have bike problems, its preferable to have the wind at your back for the return trip.

you would for comparable weather on the bike. Also, playing hockey on wheels or the ice is a great overall conditioner. There are leagues in most cities across the country.

Skiing

If you love snow and speed, alpine skiing is a great off-season workout. The first few times you hit the slopes do yourself a favor and take a lesson. You'll fall less and develop good habits instead of having to unlearn bad ones. For most people, downhill skiing is not the optimal workout since gravity is doing most of the work. Still, skiing requires strong legs, good balance, and plenty of concentration. Best of all, it's fun. Beware, it's highly addicting.

Cross-Country Skiing

It's hard to say what's the most demanding aerobic sport, but cross-country skiing is right up there. In fact, when studies are conducted on the fittest cardiovascular athletes in the world, cross-country skiers inevitably are at the top of the list. There are two styles of skiing to chose from: classic and skating. Classic, also known as diagonal stride, requires you push straight back. Skating, as the name implies, demands a skating motion. Each involves different equipment; do a lot of both and you'll get in great shape.

Snowboarding

Snowboarding is the Generation X version of skiing. Standing sideways on a board without poles, you carve turns downhill like a surfer on a wave. Snowboarding is the fastest-growing winter sport, as scores of skiers try it once and deep six their skis. Taking a lesson is very helpful since if you try and learn it on your own you're very likely to beat yourself to a pulp.

Staying Cool When It's Hot

Given a choice, we'll take summer over winter any day; however if you plan on working out regularly outside it requires some precautions, especially if you train hard or do long-distance races. Being able to wear the bare minimum when you work out is great, but exercising in the heat can be hard, even dangerous, if you are not careful.

Physiologically, the body's main objective is to make sure that the vital organs are safe. According to McArdle, Katch, and Katch's definitive textbook *Exercise Physiology*, the body can sweat as much as 3.5 liters per hour during exercise to prevent overheating. While we spoke a fair bit about what to wear when you work out in the cold, don't ignore your exercise attire on hot days. Natural fibers such as cotton soak up sweat like a sponge, so if you're out for a long workout go with synthetic fibers or risk becoming a moving puddle. For more information on garments that wick moisture away from the skin, see Chapter 23, "The Workout Wardrobe."

Another good idea is to wear light colors since they reflect heat away from the body, whereas dark colors absorb heat.

A serious concern about working out in hot weather is dehydration. It's as basic as this: As the body works to keep cool, you sweat. That means you must continue to replenish fluids. If you don't, loss of fluid volume occurs as you lose more fluid than you take in. When this happens, you stop sweating and the possibility of suffering heat illness increases. Heat illness is to summer what frostbite is to winter. The signs of heat stress are thirst, fatigue, grogginess, and visual disturbance. If these signs are ignored, heat illness can result.

There are three types of heat illness. In order of severity they are …

- ➤ Heat cramps.
- ➤ Heat exhaustion.
- ➤ Heatstroke.

Let's take a look at the symptoms and what to do about them.

Heat Cramps

Heat cramps or involuntary muscle spasms occur during or after intense exercise and afflict the muscles that are working the most intensely. (Did anyone say calf muscle?) Prevention can be assured by drinking ample amounts of water or by drinking an *electrolyte* replacement drink such as Gatorade during physical activity.

Heat Exhaustion

Symptoms of heat exhaustion are …

- ➤ A weak, rapid pulse.
- ➤ Low blood pressure while sitting.
- ➤ Headache.
- ➤ Dizziness.
- ➤ Weakness.

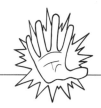

Stop Short

Even lounging around in hot weather requires special care. When you're planning on hanging out at the beach, sunscreen is a must. However, many people head out the door for a run and don't think twice about using it. Obviously exposure to the sun isn't any less when you're working out, so make sure you wear sunscreen whenever you plan to be outdoors for long periods of time. Wearing a baseball cap with a bill will also help to keep the sun off of your face. This will help decrease your exposure to damaging ultraviolet rays.

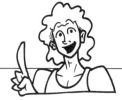

Workout Words

Electrolytes are minerals—sodium, calcium, and potassium—found in your body. When you sweat, you lose electrolytes and disturb the body's chemical composition. Drinking a fitness drink ensures you replenish these important minerals.

If you are suffering from heat exhaustion, sweating is slightly reduced but the body temperature is not elevated to dangerous levels. If you experience any of these symptoms while exercising, stop immediately and get out of the heat and drink water.

Heatstroke

Heatstroke is by far the most serious heat illness. Immediate medical attention is warranted. When heatstroke hits you, you stop sweating, the skin becomes dry and hot and the body temperature can rise to dangerous levels of 106°F and higher. This is a medical emergency and death can result if not treated quickly and correctly. While awaiting medical treatment, it is important that steps be taken to lower the core temperature with ice packs, alcohol rubs, and immersion in cold water.

While people take extra precautions when the thermometer soars, special care should also be heeded when the level of humidity is high. High humidity reduces evaporation, which prevents the body from cooling off. When this happens, your core body temperature increases, which is what can set off heat illness. When exercising in the heat, be sure to wear light colors, drink plenty of fluids (namely water), and watch the humidity.

Summer Sweatin'

There are countless sports to enjoy in the summer. As long as you take the safety precautions that we outlined above, working out in the summer is the highlight of most weekend warriors' year. Below is a sampling of some of the most popular activities that you might consider.

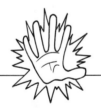

Stop Short

If you are going to swim outdoors, make sure you swim with a buddy or follow the shoreline so that you can deal with any unexpected problem and be close enough to shore. Open water swimming is a skill you need to master, so take all the necessary precautions to learn what you're doing.

Swimming

Swimming is one of the best total-body, low-impact sports that you can do—plus if you swim in a lake or the ocean, there's nothing better on a hot day. Being a "lifetime" activity, it's great for older athletes who have trouble with osteoarthritis or osteoporosis. And there are few sports better for people recovering from injuries.

If you're swimming in a lake or the ocean, the equipment requirements are pretty basic: goggles and swimsuit. People who log lots of water time often wear earplugs to prevent infections. Some people also wear nose plugs but they shouldn't be necessary if you learn how to breathe properly. Unless you are trying out for a cameo on *Baywatch*, wear a functional swimsuit, not some miniscule see-through garment that will have you meeting people you might not want to meet.

The pool is not only for swimming. Nonswimmers can participate in water aerobics classes that can be just as challenging as those done on land. One of our friends, a top New York City female runner, has been rehabbing a chronic foot injury by taking Doug Stern's Deep Water running classes. Even though she's not "running" (at least on dry land), the training sessions enable her to maintain her streak of triathlon victories.

There are also water aerobic classes, which consist of choreographed exercise routines taught by an instructor. Seen from poolside, in these classes everyone seems to be moving in slow motion; however, since every body part is exercised, these classes provide a considerable amount of resistance as you kick or push against it. Try one before you say they're not for you. Again, this is a great way to rehab an injury.

If you never learned how to swim, you can still benefit from a good workout in the pool. By using a kick board, you can use your legs to propel you through the water as you hold the kick board in front of you. If you prefer to get in an upper-body workout, use pool buoys. They fit in between your legs to hold you up as you use your arms to make your way across the pool. These workouts are deceptively hard; 15 to 20 minutes in the beginning will have you huffing and puffing. Don't believe us; try it.

Running

In the September 2000 issue of *Outside* magazine, Bernd Heinrich, a biologist and ultradistance runner, writes: "We were all runners once. Although some of us forget that primal fact, comparative biology teaches us that life on the plains generates arms races between predators and prey ...." In the mid-'70s, marathoners were considered eccentrics, but since the "running boom" exploded almost two decades ago, so many people do these races that it can be more challenging to get into big marathons like New York than to finish the race. While sneakers and clothing have become more sophisticated (and expensive), it is still the "purest" sport there is. All you need are a pair of sneakers, shorts, and T-shirt and you're good to go. In fact, though we don't recommend it, there are runners who run barefoot.

Though we've made the point before, when you run in hot weather remember the basics:

1. Drink plenty of fluids before you hit the pavement. If you start out thirsty you're bargaining for trouble during the run.

2. Wear sunblock. The sun doesn't know whether you're running in the park or lying on the beach.

3. Wear a cap to keep the sun off of your face.

4. Respect the weather. If your prerun plan is to do a track workout and it's 90°F and humid, consider postponing that workout for a less rigorous workout or just bag it and run indoors on a treadmill.

5. Try to run early in the morning before the sun's rays are strongest or late in the afternoon when the sun is less intense. The sun's rays are strongest between the hours of noon and 3 P.M.

In-Line Skating

In-line skating (also frequently called by the brand name Rollerblading) came on strong in the early 1990s. These days it seems as if everybody is doing it, from the fearless kids who jump curbs effortlessly to their grandmothers who want a low-impact workout that's also fun. It's great exercise and a great way to get around town. When you start, however, you need to practice far from motorized traffic. Learn the basics, get confident on flat, traffic-free pavement, and you're in store for years of fun.

Remember these basic safety precautions:

1. Wear a helmet. We often see skaters on the street wearing wrist guards but no helmet. If you fall and hit your head, your wrists aren't going to be good for too much.

2. Wear wrist guards. We're not saying you'll fall, but if you do, you will more than likely fall forward on outstretched hands. If you're wearing a wrist guard you're likely to damage nothing more than your pride. Without them, serious hand injuries can occur.

3. Don't wear headphones in traffic. The possibilities for accidents are too numerous.

Cycling

Back when we were kids, cycling was rather simple: You had a 10-speed racing bike, a three-speed your mom rode, and banana seat bikes for the younger set. These days, you have mountain bikes, road bikes, hybrids, BMX bikes, and recumbent bikes. Your choice of bike depends on your goals. Here's a brief synopsis on two-wheelers.

Mountain Bikes

These heavy, fat, knobby-tired bikes have changed the bike industry. Since they first appeared on the scene in the mid-'80s, mountain bikes have improved dramatically. Front and rear suspension have made riding off-road much more comfortable and safe. Many people ride mountain bikes with slick tires on the road because they're more comfortable, safer, and require less maintenance than road bikes. Jonathan, an experienced road cyclist, decided to buy a mountain bike to get to and from work. A fan of multisport races, he entered an off-road biathlon (run/bike/run) having ridden off-road a grand total of one time. Despite his prowess on the road, he knew he'd made a mistake when a woman walking her dog passed him on a gentle hill. (And they were both going down the hill.)

From a workout point of view, riding off-road provides a great workout. Riding up even a short hill spikes your heart rate, and the concentration that the sport requires is great for your head. In terms of time spent, mountain biking offers greater benefits than riding on the road.

Road Bikes

Road bikes are light (often under 20 pounds) and best ridden on a smooth surface. Since they react like a finicky poodle to anything—sand, rocks, potholes—they make poor commuter bikes. While most racing bikes cost well into four figures, you can find reliable, entry-level machines for $500 to $700.

Hybrids

As the name implies, hybrids combine the best of mountain and road bikes. They make great commuter bikes since they are lighter than mountain bikes and sturdier than road bikes. For those of you who commute to and from work on a bike, hybrids are often the best choice.

Getting out of the gym and using sporting activities to help your fitness is a great way to avoid monotony and actually have fun. Extreme conditions require a little planning to avoid discomfort or danger, but with a little attention, your outdoor workouts can be a blast.

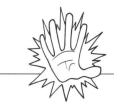

Stop Short

When you first take your nifty mountain bike off-road, do so on trails that thrill not threaten to kill you. Avoid tough single-track trails or steep descents until you're more experienced. And remember, always ride with a friend.

The Least You Need to Know

➤ Cross-training is a great way to stay fit and enjoy the seasons.

➤ If you exercise in hot or cold weather, know how to dress, how to stay hydrated, and what the warning signs of overexposure to hot and cold are.

➤ Swimming is not only for swimmers. Water aerobics and floatation devices ensure that everyone can enjoy the water.

➤ Running, cycling, blading, and swimming are potentially dangerous if you are not careful. Don't risk injury by going without proper equipment.

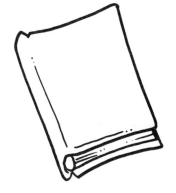

Glossary

abdominals (abs)   Muscles of the midsection.

abductors   Muscles responsible for moving the leg away from the body.

adductors   Muscles responsible for moving the leg toward the body.

barbell   A straight free weight, onto which plates can be added for resistance.

bench press (chest press)   An exercise that involves lying on your back and pushing weight from your chest.

biceps   Muscle in front of the upper arm that flexes (bends) the elbow.

body mass index (BMI)   A simple calculation that examines your weight relative to your height.

cardiovascular exercise   Any activity that involves strengthening your heart, lungs, and circulatory system.

carpal tunnel syndrome (CTS)   A condition caused by repetitive movements done with improper body mechanics, such as typing with your wrists in an extended position or repetitive squeezing activities. The median nerve swells and is unable to pass comfortably through the small bones of your wrist (carpals). Symptoms include numbness, tingling, or a sharp, shooting pain into your hand.

cartilage   Connective tissue; one of its functions is to provide covering for the ends of articular surfaces of bone, for example, between the femur (long bone of the upper thigh) and the tibia (smaller bone of the lower leg). Arthritis is the absence of cartilage between these surfaces.

circadian rhythm   Body rhythm pertaining to events that occur at approximately 24-hour intervals, such as certain physiological phenomena.

concentric contraction   Shortening of a muscle as it exerts force.

cortisol   A hormone released by the adrenal cortex. It is closely related to cortisone in its physiological effects as an anti-inflammatory.

cross-training   A training method that involves the use of a variety of exercises rather than one. For example, a runner might cross-train by using a cross-country ski machine or cycling once a week.

deltoids   The major muscle of the shoulder. Divided into the anterior (front), medial (mid), and posterior (rear) aspects.

dumbbells   Hand-held free weights.

eccentric contraction   Lengthening of the muscle as it exerts force but is overcome by the resistance.

electrolytes   Minerals—sodium, chlorine, and potassium—found in your body. When you sweat, you lose electrolytes and disturb the body's chemical composition. Fitness drinks such as Gatorade replenish these important minerals.

endorphins   Chemical substances produced in the brain that produce feelings of well-being and reduce pain.

epicondylitis   Inflammation of the tendons that attach to epicondyle bone.

ergometer   A tool for measuring the amount of work done by the user.

ergonomics   The process concerned with how to fit a job to the human body taking into account anatomical and physiological characteristics in a way that enhances human efficiency and well-being.

extend   To increase the angle between body parts, as in straightening the elbow or knee.

fartlek   A Swedish word that literally means "speed play." Fartlek workouts incorporate unstructured periods of bursts of speed. Fartlek workouts are a form of interval training.

flex   To decrease the angle between body parts, as in bending the elbow or knee (commonly, but incorrectly, used to refer to contracting a muscle).

gastrocnemius   Muscle in the back of the lower leg, responsible for raising the heel over the toe when the leg is straight.

gluteus (glutes)   Generally refers to the gluteus maximus (the gluteus medius and minimus are much smaller and weaker) responsible for extension of the hip.

hamstrings   The muscles in the back of the upper leg, responsible for bending the knee and extending the hip. Made up of the biceps femoris, semitendeinosus, and semimembranosus muscles.

heat cramps   Painful spasms of voluntary muscles following hard work in a hot environment without adequate fluid and salt intake.

heat exhaustion   An acute reaction to heat exposure. The person afflicted suffers weakness, dizziness, nausea, headache, and finally collapse.

heatstroke   An acute and dangerous reaction to heat exposure. It is characterized by high body temperature, usually above 106°F; perspiration stops, headache, numbness, tingling, and confusion occur before sudden delirium or coma.

herniation   Development of a hernia. Usually refers to a vertebral disk in the spine.

hypertension   High blood pressure.

iliotibial band   A thick band of tissue that originates from the outer part of the hip and inserts on the outer part of the knee. Iliotibial band syndrome, a common injury among runners, is a tightness that results in pain on the outer part of the leg, most likely at the knee.

impingement syndrome   The pinching or squeezing of the internal structures of the shoulder (tendons of the rotator cuff, bursa, ligaments, and nerves). This pinching causes pain on elevation of the arm.

interval training   Working out at varying levels of high and low intensity. Interval training is one of the most effective ways to increase your physiological capabilities.

isolation exercise   A lift that uses only one joint and therefore focuses on one muscle.

jet lag   Mental and physical fatigue that results from overseas flights that cover several time zones.

Karvonen method   A formula for calculating target heart rate, or training zone, that takes your resting heart rate into account.

Kegel exercise   An exercise developed by A. H. Kegel, a U.S. physician, that strengthens the pelvic wall muscles (the muscles responsible for controlling the flow of urine).

latissimus dorsi (lats)   The large, fan-shaped muscles of the middle and upper back.

manual resistance exercise   A system of strengthening exercises that use the resistance of another person instead of weights.

melatonin   Hormone produced by the pineal gland, which is responsible for making you sleepy.

obliques   Lateral abdominal muscles most responsible for rotating and flexing the trunk.

osteoporosis   Disease that results in the reduction of bone mass.

overtraining   A phenomenon that occurs when you exercise excessively without allowing sufficient recovery between workouts. Overtraining can lead to injuries and illness.

pectorals (pecs)   The large muscles of the chest.

phlebitis   An inflammation of a vein.

postpartum   Occuring after childbirth.

pronation   Turning the palms so they face palm down. In relation to the foot, it means to walk on the inner portion of your foot.

quadriceps (quads)   Muscles of the front of the upper leg, responsible for straightening the knee. Made up of the rectus femoris, vastus lateralis, vastus intermedius, and vastus medialis muscles.

range of motion (ROM)   The movement from the beginning to the finishing point of an exercise. Moving a joint from complete extension to complete flexion is considered full range of motion.

repetitive stress injury (RSI)   An injury caused by overusing muscles during repetitive activities. Commonly affects the neck, shoulder, and elbow.

resistance bands   Large, colored rubber bands of varied resistance that are used for strengthening.

resting heart rate (RHR)   Your heart rate before getting out of bed. Variations in RHR can indicate a change in conditioning or overtraining.

soleus   Muscle in the back of the lower leg, below the gastrocnemius. It is responsible for raising the heel over the toes when the leg is bent.

spin class   A group class geared toward cycling. The bikes are specially designed to provide variable levels of resistance and don't allow you to coast.

split routine   A workout scheme in which the body is divided into different parts that are exercised on different days.

spot reduction   A disproved theory that suggests that fat can be reduced in specific area of the body, for example the hips and thighs or the stomach.

supination   Turning the hand so that the palm faces upward. In relation to the foot, it means to walk on the outer portion of the foot.

target heart rate (THR)   The desired heart-rate range to elicit a training effect while performing cardiovascular exercise.

trapezius (traps)   The muscle that covers the rear aspect of the neck and shoulders.

triceps   The muscle in the back of the upper arm, responsible for straightening (extending) the elbow.

Valsalva maneuver   Holding the breath while lifting. May lead to extreme changes in blood pressure and decrease in blood returning to the heart.

vasodilator   A nerve or drug that enlarges, or dilates, the blood vessels.

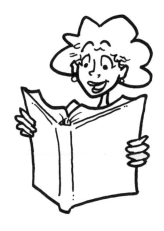

Resource Guide

Aerobics and Fitness Association of America (AFAA)
15250 Ventura Boulevard
Sherman Oaks, CA 91403
1-800-225-AFAA
www.afaa.com

American College of Sports Medicine (ACSM)
P.O. Box 1440
Indianapolis, IN 46206-1440
317-637-9200
www.acsm.org

American Council on Exercise (ACE)
5820 Oberlin Drive
Suite 102
San Diego, CA 92121-3787
1-800-825-3636
www.acefitness.org

The American Lung Association
1740 Broadway
New York, NY 10019
212-315-8700
www.lungusa.org

AquaBell

115 Marin Valley Drive

Novato, CA 94949

1-800-987-6892

www.metro.net/aquabells

BodyTrends

6385-B Rose Lane

Carpinteria, CA 93013

1-800-549-1667

www.bodytrends.com

BOWFLEX

2200 NE 65th Avenue

Vancouver, WA 98661

1-800-269-3539

www.bowflex.com

Concept II

105 Industrial Park Drive

Morrisville, VT 05661-9727

1-800-245-5676

www.concept2.com

DeSoto Sport

5260 Eastgate Mall

San Diego, CA 92121

858-453-6672

www.desotosport.com

Healthclubs.com Guide to Health and Fitness

www.healthclubs.com

International Health, Racquet & Sportsclub Association (IHRSA)

263 Summer Street

Boston, MA 02210

www.ihrsa.org

Leisure Sports Accessories, Inc. (bicycle baby seats)
18846 SE Old Trail Drive West
Jupiter, FL 33478
1-888-333-8118
www.leisuresports.com

LifeFitness
10601 West Belmont Avenue
Franklin Park, IL 60131
1-800-735-3867
www.lifefitness.com

National Sports Performance Association (NSPA)
700 Russell Avenue
Gaithersburg, MD 20877
1-800-494-6772
www.nspainc.com

Pearl Izumi
620 Compton Street
Broomfield, CO 80020
1-800-328-8488
www.pearlizumi.com

Polar Heart Rate Monitors
370 Crossways Park Drive
Woodbury, NY 11797
1-800-227-1314
www.polarusa.com

Power Blocks
Intellbell
1819 South Cedar Avenue
Owatonna, MN 55060
1-800-446-5215
www.powerblock.com

SOLOFLEX
Hawthorn Farm Industrial Park
570 NE 53rd Avenue
Hillsboro, OR 97124-6494
1-800-547-8802
www.soloflex.com

StairMaster
12421 Willows Road NE
Suite 100
Kirkland, WA 98034
1-800-635-2936
www.stairmaster.com

Strollercize
1-800-Y-STROLL
www.strollercize.com

Sweat It Out
401 West Walnut Street
P.O. Box 254
Perkasie, PA 18944
1-800-343-8960
www.sweatitout.com

Total Gym
1-800-541-4900
www.totalgym.com

U.S. Food and Drug Administration (FDA)
5600 Fishers Lane
Rockville, MD 20857
1-888-INFO-FDA (463-6332)
www.fda.gov

Index

Symbols

15-minute cardiovascular workouts
    circuit training, 108-109
    jumping rope, 104-107
    power walking, 103-104
    stair climbing, 107-108
15-minute strength-training workouts
    calisthenics, 120-123
    crunches, 115
    manual resistance exercises, 116-120
    resistance bands, 111-114
    reverse crunches, 116
30-minute cardiovascular workouts
    bike riding, 128-129
    cross-training, 130-132
    interval training, 126
    running, 126-128
    spinning, 129-130
30-minute strength-training workouts
    back raises, 144-145
    bench presses, 138-139
    chest presses, 138-139
    dips, 139-140
    lateral pull downs, 135, 137
    leg curls, 145-146
    leg extensions, 147-148
    leg presses, 134-135
    lower body workouts, 145
    seated biceps curls, 142
    shoulder presses, 141
    triceps push downs, 143
    upper body workouts, 133-134
    upright rows, 137
45-minute cardiovascular workouts, 163
    bike riding, 162
    cross-country ski machines, 164-165
    elliptical trainers, 163-164
    rowing machines, 162-163
    running, 159-162
45-minute strength-training workouts
    lower body workouts, 172-173
        abductors, 175
        adductors, 176

squats, 173-174
        standing calf raises, 177
    split routines, 178-179, 183
        concentration curls, 186
        decline presses, 180-181
        dumbbell rows, 183-184
        incline presses, 179
        shrugs, 185
        triceps kickbacks, 182
    upper-body workouts, 167-168
        flyes, 168-169
        lateral raises, 170-171
        oblique crunches, 171
45-minute total body workouts, 152
    cardiovascular, 154-155
    cool downs, 155-156
    strength-training, 157
    stretching, 156-157
    warm-ups, 152-154
60-minute cardiovascular workouts
    bike riding, 201-203
    classes, 204-205
    having fun, 206
    running, 198-201
60-minute strength-training workouts
    full-body workouts, 208-209
    lower body emphasis routines, 211-212
    push/pull split routines, 212-215
        French curls, 217-218
        front raises, 215
        reverse flyes, 216
        standing biceps curls, 213
    upper-body emphasis routines, 209-211
60-minute total body workouts, 190
    cardiovascular, 190-193
    strength-training, 193-194
    stretching, 194

A

abdominal exercises
    60-minute total body workouts, 194
    crunches, 115

mothers after pregnancy, 92
    reverse crunches, 116
abductors, 45-minute strength-training workouts, 175
ACE (American Council on Exercise), 301
ACSM (American College of Sports Medicine), 56-57, 301
activity management, 16-18
adductors, 45-minute strength-training workouts, 176
adrenaline, 8
aerobic exercise, 56-57
    classes, 63
    dress codes, 281
    THR (target heart rate), 58-59
after dark routines, tips, 20-21
after work workouts, 20-21
air temperature
    summer workouts, 290-292
    winter workouts, 288-289
altitude, workouts, 257-258
American College of Sports Medicine. See ACSM
American Council on Exercise. See ACE
American Lung Association, 131-132, 301
ankle weights, 284-285
appearance, 37
appetizers, dining out, 46-51
AquaBell, 302
    Ankle Weight Water System, 285
    Dumbbell Water System, 284
assisted living (elderly), strength training, 68-69
asthma, 30-31
    attacks, winter workouts, 289
    workout cautions, 30-31
avoiding injuries, stretching, 77-78

B

babies
    equipment
        joggers, 98
        seats, 96
        trailers, 97-98

mothers getting back into
shape, 90-92
postpartum classes, 93
strength-training, 92-93
strollercizing, 93
baby-sitting, health clubs, 95
back exercises
extensions, 269
raises, 30-minute strength-
training workouts, 144-145
seated rows, 113
stretching, 77-80, 83
bad weather, workouts, 258-259
barbell bent rows, pitfalls, 230
base layers, workout clothes,
279-280
bench presses
30-minute strength-training
workouts, 138-139
form, pitfalls, 228-229
beverages, dining out, 46-51
biceps curls
pitfalls, 232-233
resistance bands, 113
seated, 30-minute strength-
training workouts, 142
standing, 60-minute strength-
training workouts, 213
bicycle seats, 129
bike riding, 239. *See also* cycling
30-minute cardiovascular
workouts, 128-129
45-minute cardiovascular
workouts, 162
60-minute cardiovascular
workouts, 201-202
century rides, training, 202-203
hybrids, 295
mountain bikes, 294-295
road bikes, 295
bikes
45-minute total body workouts, 154
conventional upright,
60-minute total body workouts, 191-193
recumbent, 60-minute total
body workouts, 191-193
RevMaster, 204
Schwinn Air Dyne, 153
stationary
45-minute cardiovascular
workouts, 162
Lifecycle hill profile, 155
BMI (Body Mass Index), 33-34
body composition measurements,
BMI, 33-34
Body Mass Index. *See* BMI
BodyTrends, 302

bras, sports, 277
breads, carbohydrates, 44
breathing, 77
burning calories, weight loss, 39

C

calcium, dairy products, 45-46
calf raises, 271
seated, 60-minute strength-
training workouts, 208-209
standing, 45-minute strength-
training workouts, 177
calisthenics, 272
15-minute strength-training
workouts, 120-123
chin-ups, 121-122
chair dips, 273
exercises, 70-71
lunges, 122
pull-ups, 121-122
push-ups, 272
routines, 123
traveling workouts, 253
calories
burning, weight loss, 39
metabolisms, 67
calves, stretching, 85-86
canoes, paddling, 246-247
Capilene, 280
carbohydrates, 44
cardiorespiratory fitness, ACSM,
56-57
Cardiosport, heart rate monitor,
59-60
cardiovascular exercises, 56
aerobics, 56-57
body systems, 38-39, 56
children, 94
cross-training, minitriathlon,
236-237
cycling, 236-239
elliptical trainers, 236-237
endurance, fitness level, 31-32
equipment, 61, 94
fitness testing, 35-36
frequently asked questions,
56-57
goals, 56-57
golf, 241-242
health benefits, 22-23
martial arts, 245-246
meals, 61
men's norms per age groups, 36
MHR (maximum heart rate)
calculations, 58-59
motivation, 56-57
nonimpact, 236-237

paddling, 246-247
partners, 94
pitfalls, 222
StairMaster cheating, 222
treadmill cheating, 222-223
RHR (resting heart rate) calculations, 58-59
running, 236-237
skating, 242-243
skiing, 244-245
snowboarding, 244-245
spin classes, 62
step aerobics, 63
strengthening, 23-24, 56
tennis, 239, 241
THR (target heart rate), 58-59
training, 38-39
values-based prioritizing, 24-25
women's norms per age
groups, 36
workouts, 22-23
carpal tunnel syndrome. *See* CTS
cautions
asthma, workouts, 30-31
eating out, 46-51
nutritional supplements, 51-52
century rides, training, 202-203
cereal bars, 51
ceritified instructors, aerobic
classes, 63
chair dips, office workouts, 273
chairs, posture, 264-265
chest presses
30-minute strength-training
workouts, 138-139
resistance bands, 113
child care, health clubs, 95
children
mothers, 95-96
partners, cardiovascular, 94
chin tucks, 268-269
chin-ups
15-minute strength-training
workouts, 121-122
traveling workouts, 254
Chinese foods, dining out, 46-51
cholesterol, 7
circadian rhythm, jet lag, 254-257
circuit training, 15-minute cardiovascular workouts, 108-109
classes
60-minute cardiovascular
workouts, 204-205
kickboxing, 245
postpartum, 93
spinning, 204-205, 238-239
stomp, 205
Tae-Bo, 245

clothing, 275-276
  cycling shorts, 276-277
  dress codes, 280
    gyms, 280-281
    home, 280
    traveling (on the road), 281
  layering, 279
    base layers, 279-280
    insulating layers, 280
    outer layers, 280
  material, 277
    CoolMax, 278-279
    cotton, 278
    Lycra, 278
    Spandex, 278
  running shorts, 276
  shoes, 281
    fitting your foot, 282
    matching with activities,
      282-283
  singlets, 277
  socks, 277
  sport bras, 277
  summer workouts, 290-291
  winter workouts, 288-289
    ice-skating, 289-290
    in-line skating, 289-290
computers, setting up workstations, 265-266
Compu Trainer, cycling, 238-239
concentration curls, 45-minute
  strength-training workouts, 186
Concept II (C2) rowers, 152-153,
  302
  45-minute cardiovascular
    workouts, 162-163
  intervals, 155
contract/relax techniques, 273
conventional upright bikes, 60-
  minute total body workouts,
  191-193
cool downs
  45-minute total body workouts, 155-156
  60-minute total body workouts, 192
cortisol, 8
cramps, heat, 291
cross-country ski machines, 154
  45-minute cardiovascular
    workouts, 164-165
  45-minute total body workouts, 153
  60-minute total body workouts, 190-191
cross-country skiing, 290

cross-training
  30-minute cardiovascular
    workouts, 130-132
  cardiovascular, tennis, 239-241
  skating, 242-243
  triathlons, 130-132
crunches, 226
  15-minute strength-training
    workouts, 115-116
  45-minute strength-training
    workouts, 171
  oblique, 177
  pitfalls, 225-226
  resistance bands, 114
  reverse, 116
CTS (carpal tunnel syndrome),
  exercises, 262-263
curls
  biceps
    pitfalls, 232-233
    resistance bands, 113
    seated, 142
    standing, 213
  concentration, 45-minute
    strength-training workouts,
    186
  French, 60-minute strength-
    training workouts, 217-218
  legs, 30-minute strength-
    training workouts, 145-146
  seated biceps, 30-minute
    strength-training workouts,
    142
  standing biceps, 60-minute
    strength-training workouts,
    213
cycling, 239, 294. *See also* bike
  riding
  30-minute cardiovascular
    workouts, 128-130
  CompuTrainer, 238-239
  dress codes, 281
  hybrids, 295
  mountain bikes, 294-295
  road bikes, 295
  shorts, 276-277
  spinning classes, 62, 129-130,
    238-239
  stretching, 238-239
  workouts, 238-239
cyclists
  baby seats, 96
  baby trailers, 97-98
  equipment, 95-98
  mothers, training, 95-96
  spinning classes, 62, 129-130,
    238-239
  training for a century ride,
    202-203

D

daily activities and routines
  organization, 16-18
  strength-training, improvements, 68
  workouts, 16-18
dairy products, 45-46
dangers, nutritional supplements,
  51-52
decline presses, 45-minute
  strength-training workouts,
  180-181
deficiencies, vitamins and minerals, 51-52
dehydration, 291
  jet lag, 255
  water, 52
DeSoto Sport, 276, 302
desserts, dining out, 46-51
desynchronosis, 254-257
detraining, workouts, 40
developing habits, workouts, 9
diabetes
  BMI, 33-34
  medical conditions, 29-30
dieting, feeling healthy, 37
dining out, 46-51
dips
  30-minute strength-training
    workouts, 139-140
  chair, calisthenics, 273
disorientation, jet lag, 255
double leg lifts, pitfalls, 227-228
downhill skiing, 290
dress codes, workout clothes,
  280-281
drinking fluids, jet lag, 256
dumbbell rows, 45-minute
  strength-training workouts,
  183-184
DynaBands, 15-minute strength-
  training workouts, 111-114

E

eating out, cautions, 46-51
elderly assisted living, strength-
  training, 68-69
electrolytes, replacing, 291
elliptical trainers
  45-minute cardiovascular
    workouts, 163-164
  60-minute total body workouts, 190-192
  cardiovascular exercise,
    236-237

endorphins, workouts, 10
entrées, dining out, 46-51
equipment
    baby joggers, 98
    baby trailers, 97-98
    BOWFLEX, 71-73
    cardiovascular, 94
    Cybex, 71-73
    cyclist, 95-96
    free weights, 73
    home gyms, 71-73
    Nautilus, 71-73
    PowerBlock, 73
    SOLOFLEX, 71-73
    workouts, 71-73
essential nutrients, 41-42
excuses for not working out, 14
exercises, 163. *See also* fitness;
  workouts
    abdominals, 92
    calisthenics, 70-71, 253, 272
        chair dips, 273
        chin-ups, 254
        pull-ups, 254
        push-ups, 253-254, 272
    cardiovascular, 154-155, 163,
      190-193, 206
        bike riding, 128-129, 162,
          201-203
        circuit training, 108-109
        classes, 62, 204-205
        Concept II (C2) rower
          intervals, 155
        cross-country ski machines,
          164-165
        cross-training, 130-132
        cycling, 238-239
        elliptical trainers, 163-164
        golf, 241-242
        interval training, 126
        jumping rope, 104-107, 253
        Lifecycle hill profile, 155
        martial arts, 245-246
        paddling, 246-247
        pitfalls, 222-223
        power walking, 103-104
        rowing machines, 162-163
        running, 126-128, 159-162,
          198-201, 236-237
        skating, 242-243
        skiing, 244-245
        snowboarding, 244-245
        spinning, 129-130, 204-205
        stair climbing, 107-108
        StairMaster Lunar Landing
          program, 155
        stomping classes, 205
        tennis, 239, 241
    children, 94
    contract/relax techniques, 273

cool downs, 155-156
feeling healthy, 37
gluteals, 93
habits, 9
high altitudes, 257-258
Kegel, 92
multi-joint, 134
muscle groups, 69
parents, 94
physiological effects, 38
postpartum classes, 93
stair workouts, 271-272
strength and endurance, 34-35
strength training, 69, 94-95,
  157, 193-194, 270
    abductors, 175
    adductors, 176
    back raises, 144-145
    bench presses, 138-139
    calf raises, 271
    calisthenics, 120-121, 123
    chest presses, 138-139
    chin-ups, 121-122
    concentration curls, 186
    crunches, 115, 226
    decline presses, 180-181
    dips, 139-140
    dumbbell rows, 183-184
    flyes, 168-169
    forearm extensions, 270
    forearm flexions, 271
    French curls, 217-218
    front raises, 215
    full-body workouts, 208
    gluteus squeezes, 271
    hamstring squeezes, 271
    incline presses, 179
    lateral pull downs, 135-137
    lateral raises, 170-171
    leg curls, 145-146
    leg emphasis, 157, 193
    leg extensions, 147-148
    leg presses, 134-135
    lower-body workouts, 145,
      172-173, 211-212
    lunges, 122
    manual resistance exercises,
      116-120
    oblique crunches, 171
    pitfalls, 225-233
    pull-ups, 121-122
    push-ups, 121
    push/pull split routines,
      212-215
    quadriceps squeezes, 271
    resistance bands, 111-114,
      254
    reverse crunches, 116
    reverse flyes, 216

scapula retractions, 270
seated biceps curls, 142
seated calf raises, 208-209
shoulder presses, 141
shrugs, 185
split routines, 178-179, 183
squats, 173-174
standing biceps curls, 213
standing calf raises, 177
triceps kickbacks, 182
triceps push downs, 143
upper-body workouts,
  133-134, 157, 167-168,
  193, 210-211
upright rows, 137
stress management, 8
stretching, 156-157, 194, 267
    back extensions, 269
    chin tucks, 268-269
    levator scapula stretches,
      267
    pitfalls, 223-225
    side stretches, 269
    trapizius stretches, 267
strollercizing, 93
traveling, 283-284
warm-ups, 152-154
workout partners, 94
exhaustion, heat, 291-292
extensions
    back, 269
    forearm, 270
    legs, 30-minute strength-
      training workouts, 147-148
    triceps, resistance bands, 113

F

fabrics, workout clothes, 278
fartlek, 127
fast foods, dining out, 46-51
fatigue, jet lag, 255
FDA (U.S. Food and Drug
  Administration), 304
feeling healthy, 37
finger stretches, 262-263
fitness. *See also* exercises; workouts
    apperances, 37
    cardiovascular testing, 35-36
    flexibility, 31-32, 36
    goals, 31-32
    levels, 31-32
    measurement, 27-28
    mothers, 95-96
    obstacles, 5-7
    safety, 27-28
    strengthening, 31-35
    tests, 34-36

fleece, 280
flexibility
  fitness level, 31-32
  stretching, 24, 36
  testing, 36
flexions, forearm, 271
flyes
  45-minute strength-training
    workouts, 168-169
  reverse, 60-minute strength-
    training workouts, 216
Food Guide Pyramid, 43, 46
forearms
  extensions, 270
  flexions, 271
  stretches, 262
free weights, equipment, 73
French curls, 60-minute strength
  training workouts, 217-218
frequency, strength-training,
  69-70
frequently asked questions,
  cardiovascular exercise, 56-57
front raises
  60-minute strength training
    workouts, 215
  resistance bands, 113
fruit juices, 51
fruits, 44
full-body strength-training workouts, 60-minutes, 208-209
fuzziness, jet lag, 255

G

gluteals
  exercises, mothers after preg-
    nancy, 93
  squeezes, 271
goals
  fitness level, 31-32
  setting, 56-57
  workouts, 22
gold, strength-training, 241-242
golf, 241-243
good mornings, pitfalls, 230-231
Gore-Tex, 280
granola bars, 51
Gravitron, dips, 140
groin, stretching, 84
guidelines, manual resistance
  exercises, 119-120
gyms
  exercise classes, 62
  workout clothes dress codes,
    280-281

H

habits, workouts, 9
hamstrings
  squeezes, 271
  stretching, 79-80
hand presses, 263
Hawaiian Ironman, 131
health benefits
  aerobics, 56
  cardiovascular
    fitness, 22-23
    training, 38-39
  hormones, 8
  muscles, 37-38
  nutrition, 41-42
  strength training, 23-24, 37-39
  stretching, 24, 39
  vegetables, 44-45
  water, 52
  workouts, 7-11
health clubs, child care, 95
healthy eating, 37, 46-51
heart disease, BMI, 33-34
heart rate
  maximum, 58-59
  monitors, 59-60
  resting, 33
  target, 58-59
heat
  cramps, 291
  exhaustion, 291-292
  strokes, 292
  summer workouts, 290-291
high altitudes, symptoms,
  257-258
hips
  abductors, 45-minute strength-
    training workouts, 175
  flexors, 83-84
  stretching, 80, 83-84
home gym equipment, 71-73
homepathic remedies, no-jet-lag,
  257
hurdler's stretches, pitfalls, 224
hybrids, 295
hydration
  aerobic classes, 63
  water, 52
  workouts, 61
hypertension
  BMI, 33-34
  medical conditions, 29

I–K

IHRSA (International Health,
  Racquet & Sportsclub
  Association), 252, 302
Iliotibial Band Syndrome, 194
illness, running dilemmas, 199
incline presses, 45-minute
  strength-training workouts, 179
injuries
  aerobic classes, 63
  back pain, 77-78
  prevention methods, 77-78
  rehabilitation, weight-training,
    67-68
  stretching, 24, 77-78
instructions, measuring heart rate,
  33
instructors (ceritified), aerobic
  classes, 63
insulating layers, workout
  clothes, 280
International Health, Racquet &
  Sportsclub Association.
  See IHRSA
interval training, 126, 155.
  See also training
  30-minute cardiovascular
    workouts, 126
  bike riding, 162
  Concept II (C2) rower inter-
    vals, 155
  cross-country ski machines,
    164-165
  elliptical trainers, 163-164
  Lifecycle hill profile, 155
  martial arts, 245-246
  power walking to running
    programs, 128
  rowing machines, 162-163
  StairMaster Lunar Landing
    program, 155
  treadmills, 160-161
involuntary muscle spasms, 291
irrational, unreasonable behavior,
  jet lag, 255
Italian foods, dining out, 46-51

Japanese foods, dining out, 46-51
jet lag, 254-257
  circadian rhythm, 254-257
  dehydration, 255
  disorientation, 255
  drinking fluids, 256
  fatigue, 255
  fuzziness, 255

irrational, unreasonable behavior, 255
preflight, 256
sleep, 255-256
swollen legs and feet, 255
joggers equipment, baby joggers, 98
jumping rope
15-minute cardiovascular workouts, 104-105
choosing a rope, 105
type of rope, 105-107
traveling workouts, 253
junk foods, 45-46

Karvonen, THR, 58-59
kayaks, paddling, 246-247
Kegel exercises, 92
kickboxing, 245
kickbacks (triceps), 45-minute strength-training workouts, 182

L

lactose intolerant, dairy products, 45-46
laterals
epicondylitis, 240
pull downs, 30-minute strength-training workouts, 135-137
raises
45-minute strength-training workouts, 170-171
resistance bands, 113
layering
winter workouts, 288-290
workout clothes, 279
base layers, 279-280
insulating layers, 280
outer layers, 280
legs
curls, 30-minute strength-training workouts, 145-146
extensions, 30-minute strength-training workouts, 147-148
lifts, pitfalls, 231
presses
30-minute strength-training workouts, 134-135
seated, resistance bands, 113
strength-training
45-minute total body workouts, 157
60-minute total body workouts, 193

levator scapula stretches, 267
Lifecycle, 240
30-minute cardiovascular workouts, 128-129
45-minute cardiovascular workouts, 162
60-minute total body workouts, 192
hill profile, 155
LifeFitness, 303
lifestyle changes, feeling healthy, 37
lifters, manual resistance exercise guidelines, 119
lifting. *See also* strength training; weight lifting
60-minute total body workouts; 193
legs, 193
upper body, 193
abductors, 45-minute strength-training workouts, 175
adductors, 45-minute strength-training workouts, 176
back raises, 30-minute strength-training workouts, 144-145
bench presses, 30-minute strength-training workouts, 138-139
chest presses, 30-minute strength-training workouts, 138-139
circuit training, 108-109
concentration curls, 45-minute strength-training workouts, 186
decline presses, 45-minute strength-training workouts, 180-181
dips, 30-minute strength-training workouts, 139-140
dumbbell rows, 45-minute strength-training workouts, 183-184
explosively, 227
flyes, 45-minute strength-training workouts, 168-169
French curls, 217-218
front raises, 215
golf, 241-242
good mornings, 230-231
incline presses, 45-minute strength-training workouts, 179
lateral pull downs, 30-minute strength-training workouts, 135, 137

lateral raises, 45-minute strength-training workouts, 170-171
leg curls, 30-minute strength-training workouts, 145-146
leg extensions, 30-minute strength-training workouts, 147-148
leg presses, 30-minute strength-training workouts, 134-135
lifting explosively, 227
martial arts, 245-246
paddling, 246-247
pitfalls
barbell bent rows, 230
bench press form, 228-229
biceps curls, 232-233
double leg lifts, 227-228
leg lifts, 231
stiff-legged dead lifts, 230-231
reverse flyes, 216
seated biceps curls, 30-minute strength-training workouts, 142
seated calf raises, 208-209
shoulder presses, 30-minute strength-training workouts, 141
shrugs, 45-minute strength-training workouts, 185
skating, 242-243
skiing, 244-245
snowboarding, 244-245
squats, 45-minute strength-training workouts, 173-174
standing biceps curls, 213
standing calf raises, 45-minute strength-training workouts, 177
tennis, 239, 241
triceps kickbacks, 45-minute strength-training workouts, 182
triceps push downs, 30-minute strength-training workouts, 143
upright rows, 30-minute strength-training workouts, 137
loose fist presses, 263
lower body (strength-training)
30-minute workouts, 145
leg curls, 145-146
leg extensions, 147-148
45-minute workouts, 172-173
abductors, 175
adductors, 176

squats, 173-174
standing calf raises, 177
60-minute strength training workouts, 211-212
lunchtime routines, workouts, 20
lunges, 15-minute strength-training workouts, 122

M

manual resistance exercises, 15-minute strength-training workouts, 116-120
marathons, 198
training, 198-201
Web sites, 201
martial arts, 245-246
material, workout clothes, 277-279
maximum heart rate. *See* MHR
meals, 61
measurements, 27-28
measuring
fitness level, 31-32
heart rate, 33
medical conditions
asthma, 30-31
diabetes, 29-30
hypertension, 29
melatonin, 257
men
cardiovascular norms per age group, 36
push-ups norms, 34
metabolism
calories, 67
muscles, burn calories, 67
Mexican foods, dining out, 46-51
MHR (maximum heart rate), 58-59
minerals, carbohydrates, 44
minitriathlons, 236
misconceptions, muscles and strength, 37-38
Mittleman, Stu, 9
morning routines, workouts, 18-19
mothers
baby joggers, 98
baby trailers, 97-98
children, 95-96
cyclist training, 95-96
getting into shape, 90-92
postpartum classes, 93
strength-training, 92-93
strollercizing, 93

sleep deprivation, 95-96
workouts, 95-96
motivation, cardiovascular exercise, 56-57
mountain bikes, 294-295
muffins, 50
multijoint exercises, 30-minute strength-training workouts, 133-134, 145
multivitamins, nutritional supplements, 51-52
muscles
awe-inspiring, 66
descriptions, 66
exercises, 69
fitness level, 31-32
health benefits, 37-38
involuntary spasms, 291
metabolisms, burn calories, 67
misconceptions and myths, 37-38
strength-training, 31-32, 66, 69
stretching, 76-77
myths, muscles and strength, 37-38

N

National Sports Performance Association. *See* NSPA, 303
Nautilus, skating stimulators, 242
no-jet-jag, 257
nonorganics, proteins, 45
NordicTrack, 45-minute cardiovascular workouts, 164-165
not working out, excuses, 14
novices, fitness level, 31-32
NSPA (National Sports Performance Association), 303
nutrients, essential, 41-42
nutrition
dining out tips, 46-51
essential nutrients, 41-42
Food Guide Pyramid, 43
general guidelines, 43
health benefits, 41-42
junk food, 45-46
nutrients, 41-42
nuts, 50
programs, eating out, 46-51
supplements, 51-52
vegetables, 44-45
water, 52
nutritionists, recommended portions, 41-42
nuts, 50

O

oblique crunches, 45-minute strength-training workouts, 171
office posture, 263
chairs, 264-265
workstations, 265-266
office workouts
calisthenics, 272-273
contract/relax techniques, 273
stairs, 271-272
strength-training, 270
calf raises, 271
forearm extensions, 270
forearm flexions, 271
gluteus squeezes, 271
hamstring squeezes, 271
quadriceps squeezes, 271
scapula retractions, 270
stretching, 267
back extensions, 269
chin tucks, 268-269
levator scapula stretches, 267
side stretches, 269
trapizius stretches, 267
oils and fats, 44-45
organics
fruits, 44
proteins, 45
organization
daily routines, 16-18
time management, 14-17
osteoporosis, prevention techniques, 67-68
outer layers, workout clothes, 280
Overend, Ned, triathlons, 289
overtraining, 40, 161

P

paddling, 246-247
PAR Q (Physical Activity Readiness Questionnaire), 27-28
parents, exercises, 94
partners, strength-training, 94-95
Pearl Izumi, 277, 303
pectorals, stretching, 86-87
Philibim, John, 117
phlebitis, 256-257
Physical Activity Readiness Questionnaire. *See* PAR Q, 27-28
physical checkups, physicians, 27-28
physical health benefits, 11, 95-96

physical therapists
osteoporosis, 67-68
stretching, 76-77
physicians, physical checkups, 27-28
physiological effects
exercises, 38
strength-training, structure and function, 39
stretching, 39
pile, 280
pitfalls
barbell bent rows, 230
bench press form, 228-229
biceps curls, 232-233
crunches, 225-226
double leg lifts, 227-228
good mornings, 230-231
hurdler's stretches, 224
leg lifts, 231
lifting explosively, 227
resistance bands, 112
sit-ups, 231-232
StairMaster, 222
standing toe touches, 223-224
stiff-legged dead lifts, 230-231
treadmills, 222-223
workstation posture, 265
yoga, plough position, 225
Polar Heart Rate Monitors, 303
polyester microfiber, 280
polypropylene, 280
postpartum classes, exercises, 93
posture, 263
chairs, 264-265
workstations, 265-266
Power Blocks, 303
power walking, 15-minute cardiovascular workouts, 103-104
preflight, jet lag, 256
pregnancies, getting back into shape, 90-92
postpartum classes, 93
strength-training, 92-93
strollercizing, 93
presses
bench, 30-minute strength-training workouts, 138-139
chest
30-minute strength-training workouts, 138-139
resistance bands, 113
decline, 45-minute strength-training workouts, 180-181
hand, 263
incline, 45-minute strength-training workouts, 179
legs, 30-minute strength-training workouts, 134-135

loose fist, 263
seated leg, 15-minute strength-training workouts, 113
shoulder, 30-minute strength-training workouts, 141
principles, strength-training, 66
programs
century rides, 203
interval training, 155
marathon training, 200
power walking to running, 128
treadmill workouts, 127
pronate, 282
proteins, 45
psychological benefits, workouts, 10-11
pull downs (lateral), 30-minute strength-training workouts, 135-137
pull-ups
15-minute strength-training workouts, 121-122
traveling, workouts, 254
pulse, heart monitoring, 59-60
push downs (triceps), 30-minute strength-training workouts, 143
push-ups
15-minute strength-training workouts, 121
men's norms, 34
office workouts, 272
traveling workouts, 253-254
women's norms, 35
push/pull split routines, 60-minute strength training workouts, 212-215
French curls, 217-218
front raises, 215
reverse flyes, 216
standing biceps curls, 213

Q–R

quadriceps
squeezes, 271
stretching, 78-79
raises
back, 30-minute strength-training workouts, 144-145
calf, 177, 208-209, 271
front
60-minute strength-training workouts, 215
resistance bands, 113

lateral
45-minute strength-training workouts, 170-171
resistance bands, 113
seated calf, 60-minute strength-training workouts, 208-209
standing calf, 45-minute strength training workouts, 177
recommended food portions, nutritionists, 41-42
recumbent bikes, 60-minute total body workouts, 191-193
rehabilitation, weight-training injuries, 67-68
relax/contract techniques, 273
repetitive stress injury. *See* RSI
repititions, 70
resistance bands, 283-284
15-minute strength-training workouts, 111-114
biceps curls, 113
chest presses, 113
crunches, 114
front raises, 113
lateral raises, 113
reverse crunches, 114
seated leg presses, 113
seated rows, 113
triceps extensions, 113
AquaBell Dumbbell Water System, 284
pitfalls, 112
traveling workouts, 254
resistance exercises (manual), 15-minute strength-training workouts, 116-120
resistance training, weight-training, 70
restaurant portions, eating out, 46-51
resting heart rate. *See* RHR
retractions, scapula, 270
reverse crunches
15-minute strength-training workouts, 116
resistance bands, 114
reverse flyes, 60-minute strength training workouts, 216
RevMaster bikes, 204
RHR (resting heart rate), 33, 58-59
rice, carbohydrates, 44
rice cakes, 51
road bikes, 295
Rollerblading, 294
routines
after work workouts, 20-21
calisthenics, 15-minute strength-training workouts, 123

inactivity, 9-10
lower-body emphasis,
  60-minute strength-training
  workouts, 211-212
lunchtime workouts, 20
morning workouts, 18-19
push/pull split, 60-minute
  strength-training workouts,
  212-218
short workouts, 11-12
split, 45-minute strength-
  training workouts,
  178-179, 183
strength-training, 69
  lower body, 172-173
  upper body, 167-168
stretching, 45-minute total
  body workouts, 156-157
tips, 94
upper-body emphasis,
  60-minute strength-training
  workouts, 209-211
work out at work, 21
rowing machines
  45-minute cardiovascular
    workouts, 162-163
  45-minute total body work-
    outs, 153
  Concept II (C2) rowers,
    153-155
rows
  dumbbell, 45-minute strength-
    training workouts, 183-184
  seated, resistance bands, 113
  upright, 30-minute strength-
    training workouts, 137
RSI (repetitive stress injury),
  262-263
running, 293-294
  30-minute cardiovascular
    workouts, 126-128
  45-minute cardiovascular
    workouts, 159-162
  60-minute cardiovascular
    workouts, 198
  cardiovascular exercise,
    236-237
  dress codes, 281
  shorts, 276
  sickness, 199
  strength-training, 236-237
  stretching, 236-237
  training for a marathon,
    198-201
  treadmills, 126-128, 159-162
  weight-lifting, 236-237

S

safety, fitness level, 27-28
scapula retractions, 270
schedules
  marathon training program,
    200
  training for a century ride, 203
seasonal workouts
  summer, 290-292
    cycling, 294-295
    heat cramps, 291
    heat exhaustion, 291-292
    heatstrokes, 292
    in-line skating, 294
    running, 293-294
    swimming, 292-293
  winter, 288-289
    ice-skating, 289-290
    in-line skating, 289-290
    skiing, 290
    snowboarding, 290
seated biceps curls, 30-minute
  strength-training workouts, 142
seated calf rasises, 60-minute
  strength-training workouts,
  208-209
seated leg presses, resistance
  bands, 113
seated rows, resistance bands, 113
self-confidence, appearance, 37
sets and reps, 70-71
setting goals, 22, 56-57
shoes, workout clothes, 281
  fitting your foot, 282
  matching with activities,
    282-283
short workouts, 5-7, 11-12
shorts
  cycling, 276-277
  running, 276
shoulder exercises, 113
shoulder impingement syndrome,
  136
shoulder presses, 30-minute
  strength-training workouts, 141
shrugs, 45-minute strength-training
  workouts, 185
sickness, running dilemmas, 199
side stretches, 269
singlets, 277
sit-ups, pitfalls, 231-232
skating
  cardiovascular exercise, 242-243
  in-line, 294
  stretching, 242-243
  weight lifting, 242-243

skiing
  cardiovascular exercise, 244-245
  cross-country, 290
  downhill, 290
  strength-training, 244-245
  stretching, 244-245
  weight lifting, 244-245
sleep
  deprivation, mothers, 95-96
  jet lag, 255-256
snacking, between meals, 46-51
sneakers. *See* shoes
socks, 277
sodas, 50
SOLOFLEX, 304
soups, dining out, 46-51
speed of movement, lifting, 70
spinning
  30-minute cardiovascular
    workouts, 129-130
  60-minute cardiovascular
    workouts, 204-205
  classes, 62, 238-239
  dress codes, 281
split routines, 45-minute strength
  training workouts, 178-179, 183
  concentration curls, 186
  decline presses, 180-181
  dumbbell rows, 183-184
  incline presses, 179
  shrugs, 185
  triceps kickbacks, 182
sports bras, 277
sports
  cross-country skiing, 290
  cycling, 294
    hybrids, 295
    mountain bikes, 294-295
    road bikes, 295
  downhill skiing, 290
  ice-skating, 289-290
  in-line skating, 289-290, 294
  running, 293-294
  snowboarding, 290
  swimming, 292-293
spot reduction, 194
spotters, manual resistance exercise guidelines, 120
squats, 45-minute strength-training
  workouts, 173-174
squeezes, 271
stair climbing
  15-minute cardiovascular
    workouts, 107-108
  workouts, 271-272
StairMaster, 240, 304
  60-minute total body workouts,
    192
  cheating, 222

Lunar Landing program, 155
RevMaster bike, 204
stomp classes, 205
standing biceps curls, 60-minute
strength training workouts, 213
standing calf raises, 45-minute
strength-training workouts, 177
standing toe touches, pitfalls,
223-224
starchy foods, carbohydrates, 44
stationary bikes
45-minute cardiovascular
workouts, 162
45-minute total body workouts,
153
Lifecycle hill profile, 155
step aerobics, 63
steroids, proteins, 45
stiff-legged dead lifts, pitfalls,
230-231
stomp classes, 60-minute cardiovascular workouts, 205
strength
endurance exercises, 34-35
health benefits, 37-38
fitness test, 34-35
misconceptions and myths,
37-38
strength training. *See also* lifting;
weight training
cardiovascular fitness, 23-24
circuit training, 108-109
crunches, 226
daily activities, 68
dress codes, 281
elderly, assisted living, 68-69
exercises, 69, 94-95
frequency, 69-70
golf, 241-243
health benefits, 23-24, 39
lifting explosively, 227
martial arts, 245-246
mothers after pregnancy, 92-93
muscles, 66, 69
office workouts, 270-271
osteoporosis, 67-68
paddling, 246-247
partners, 94-95
physiological effects, structure
and function, 39
pitfalls, 225
barbell bent rows, 230
bench press form, 228-229
biceps curls, 232-233
crunches, 225-226
double leg lifts, 227-228
good mornings, 230-231
leg lifts, 231
sit-ups, 231-232
stiff-legged dead lifts,
230-231

principles, 66, 69
resistance exercises, 94-95
routines, 69
running, 236-237
skiing, 244-245
snowboarding, 244-245
tennis, 239, 241
weight training, 67-68
workouts, 69-71
stress management, workouts, 7-9
stretching, 77-78
45-minute total body workouts,
156-157
60-minute total body workouts,
194
avoiding injuries, 77-78
back muscles, 77-80, 83
basic stretches, 77-78
breathing, 76-77
calves, 85-86
CTS (carpal tunnel syndrome),
262-263
cycling, 238-239
flexibility, 24, 36
golf, 241-242
groin, 84
hamstrings, 79-80
health benefits, 24, 39
hip flexors, 80, 83-84
injuries, 24, 77-78
martial arts, 245-246
meditation, 76-77
muscle tightness, 76-77
office workouts, 267-269
paddling, 246-247
pectorals, 86-87
physical therapists, 76-77
physiological effects, 39
pitfalls, 223
hurdler's stretches, 224
standing toe touches,
223-224
yoga plough, 225
quadriceps, 78-79
RSI (repetitive stress injury),
262-263
running, 236-237
skating, 242-243
skiing, 244-245
snowboarding, 244-245
stair climbing, 108
tennis, 239, 241
warm-ups, 76-77
yoga, 87
strollercizing, 93, 304
structure and function, cardiovascular system, 38-39
summer, exercising, 290-292
cycling, 294-295
heat cramps, 291

heat exhaustion, 291-292
heatstrokes, 292
in-line skating, 294
running, 293-294
swimming, 292-293
supinate, 282
supplements, nutritional, 51-52
Supplex, 280
surgeries, rehabilitation, 67-68
swimming, 292-293
swollen legs and feet, jet lag, 255
symptoms, high-altitude exercises, 257-258

T

Tae-Bo, 245
target heart rate. *See* THR
teachers, spinning classes, 62
techniques, contract/relax, 273
tennis, 239-241
tennis elbow, 240
tennis shoes. *See* shoes
tensions, contract/relax techniques, 273
terminology, reps, 70
testing
cardiovascular fitness, 35-36
flexibility, 36
TheraBands, 15-minute strength-
training workouts, 111-114
therapeutic benefits, workouts,
7-8
Thermastat, 280
Thermax, 280
Thermion, 280
Thorlo, socks, 277
THR (target heart rate), 58-59
time management
activity management, 16-18
organization, 14-17
workouts, 14-18
tips
abduction, 175
adduction, 176
after dark routines, 20-21
bench presses, 139
biceps curls, 142
century rides, 202
chest presses, 139
concentration curls, 186
crunches, 115
decline presses, 181
dips, 140
dumbbell rows, 184
flyes, 169
French curls, 218
front raises, 215
incline presses, 179

jumping rope, 106
lateral pull downs, 137
lateral raises, 171
leg curls, 146
leg extensions, 147
leg presses, 135
morning routine workouts,
    18-19
oblique crunches, 171
organization, 14-17
quizzes, 5-7
reverse flyes, 216
routines, 94
seated calf raises, 209
shoulder presses, 141
shrugs, 185
squats, 174
standing biceps curls, 213
standing calf raises, 177
time management, 14-17
training for a marathon, 201
triceps kickbacks, 182
triceps push downs, 143
upright rows, 137
work out at work, 21
workstation posture, 265
toe touches (standing), pitfalls,
    223-224
training. *See also* interval training
    century rides, 202-203
    circuit, 15-minute cardiovascu-
        lar workouts, 108-109
    interval, 126, 155, 163
    marathons, 198-201
    triathlons, 130-132
trapezius stretches, 267
traveling
    dress codes, workout clothes,
        281
    jet lag, 254-257
    resistance bands, 283-284
    workouts, 252-253
        calisthenics, 253
        chin-ups, 254
        jumping rope, 253
        pull-ups, 254
        push-ups, 253-254
        resistance bands, 254
        tips, 21-22
treadmills, 159-162
    30-minute cardiovascular
        workouts, 126-128
    45-minute total body workouts,
        154
    60-minute total body workouts,
        192
    cheating, 222-223
triathlons, 130-131

triceps
    extensions, resistance bands,
        113
    kickbacks, 45-minute strength-
        training workouts, 182
    push downs, 30-minute
        strength-training workouts,
        143

U

U.S. Department of Health and
    Human Services, Food Guide
    Pyramid, 43
U.S. Food and Drug
    Administration. *See* FDA
Ultrex, 280
unhealthy snacks, 46-51
upper body (strength training)
    30-minute workouts, 133-134
        back raises, 144-145
        bench presses, 138-139
        chest presses, 138-139
        dips, 139-140
        lateral pull downs, 135-137
        leg presses, 134-135
        seated biceps curls, 142
        shoulder presses, 141
        triceps push downs, 143
        upright rows, 137
    45-minute workouts, 157,
        167-168
        flyes, 168-169
        lateral raises, 170-171
        oblique crunches, 171
    60-minute workouts, 193,
        209-211
upright rows, 30-minute strength-
    training workouts, 137

V

Valsalva maneuvers, 138
values-based prioritizing, workouts,
    24-25
vegetables, 44-45
VersaClimber, 60-minute total
    body workouts, 190-191
Vertical Challenge, triathlons,
    131-132
veterans, fitness level, 31-32
vitamins
    carbohydrates, 44
    dairy products, 45-46
    deficiencies, 51-52
    fruits, 44

megadoses, 51-52
proteins, 45
supplements (nutritional),
    51-52

W–Z

walking (power), 15-minute car-
    diovascular workouts, 103-104
wardrobe, 275-276
    ankle weights, 284-285
    cycling shorts, 276-277
    dress codes, 280-281
    layering, 279-280
    material, 277
    resistance bands, 283-284
    running shorts, 276
    shoes, 281-283
    singlets, 277
    socks, 277
    sports bras, 277
warm-ups
    45-minute total body work-
        outs, 152-154
    stretching, 76-77
water, 52
weather, workouts, 258-259
weight composition, BMI, 33-34
weight loss
    burning calories, 39
    fitness, values-based prioritiz-
        ing, 24-25
    textbook examples, 39
weight lifting. *See also* lifting;
    strength training
    60-minute total body work-
        outs, 193
    abductors, 45-minute strength-
        training workouts, 175
    adductors, 45-minute strength-
        training workouts, 176
    back raises, 30-minute
        strength-training workouts,
        144-145
    bench presses, 30-minute
        strength-training workouts,
        138-139
    chest presses, 30-minute
        strength-training workouts,
        138-139
    circuit training, 108-109
    concentration curls, 45-minute
        strength-training workouts,
        186
    decline presses, 45-minute
        strength-training workouts,
        180-181

dips, 30-minute strength-training workouts, 139-140
dumbbell rows, 45-minute strength-training workouts, 183-184
flyes, 45-minute strength-training workouts, 168-169
French curls, 217-218
front raises, 215
golf, 241-242
incline presses, 45-minute strength-training workouts, 179
lateral pull downs, 30-minute strength-training workouts, 135, 137
lateral raises, 45-minute strength-training workouts, 170-171
leg curls, 30-minute strength-training workouts, 145-146
leg extensions, 30-minute strength-training workouts, 147-148
leg presses, 30-minute strength-training workouts, 134-135
lifting explosively, 227
martial arts, 245-246
paddling, 246-247
pitfalls
    barbell bent rows, 230
    bench press form, 228-229
    biceps curls, 232-233
    double leg lifts, 227-228
    good mornings, 230-231
    leg lifts, 231
    stiff-legged dead lifts, 230-231
rehabilitation, surgeries, 67-68
repititions, 70
resistance training, 70
reverse flyes, 216
running, 236-237
seated biceps curls, 30-minute strength-training workouts, 142
seated calf raises, 208-209
shoulder presses, 30-minute strength-training workouts, 141
shrugs, 45-minute strength-training workouts, 185
skating, 242-243
skiing, 244-245
snowboarding, 244-245
squats, 45-minute strength-training workouts, 173-174
standing biceps curls, 213

standing calf raises, 45-minute strength-training workouts, 177
strength training, 67-68
tennis, 239, 241
tennis, 239, 241
triceps kickbacks, 45-minute strength-training workouts, 182
triceps push downs, 30-minute strength-training workouts, 143
upright rows, 30-minute strength-training workouts, 137
weights, ankle, 284-285
whole-grains, carbohydrates, 44
wind chill, 288-289
wind velocity, 288-289
winter, exercising, 288-289
women
    cardiovascular norms per age group, 36
    push-up norms, 35
wool, 280
work
    calisthenics, 272
        chair dips, 273
        push-ups, 272
    contract/relax techniques, 273
    stair workouts, 271-272
    strength-training, 270
        calf raises, 271
        forearm extensions, 270
        forearm flexions, 271
        gluteus squeezes, 271
        hamstring squeezes, 271
        quadriceps squeezes, 271
        scapula retractions, 270
    stretching, 267
        back extensions, 269
        chin tucks, 268-269
        levator scapula stretches, 267
        side stretches, 269
        trapezius stretches, 267
    workouts, routines, 21
workout clothes, 275-276
    cycling shorts, 276-277
    dress codes, 280-281
    layering, 279-280
    materials, 277-279
    running shorts, 276
    shoes, 281
        fitting your foot, 282
        mathching with activities, 282-283
    singlets, 277
    socks, 277
    sport bras, 277

workouts, 21. *See also* exercises; fitness
    15-minute cardiovascular
        circuit training, 108-109
        jumping rope, 104-107
        power walking, 103-104
        stair climbing, 107-108
    15-minute strength-training
        calisthenics, 120-123
        crunches, 115
        manual resistance exercises, 116-120
        resistance bands, 111-114
        reverse crunches, 116
    30-minute cardiovascular
        bike riding, 128-129
        cross-training, 130-132
        interval training, 126
        running, 126-128
        spinning, 129-130
    30-minute strength-training
        back raises, 144-145
        bench presses, 138-139
        chest presses, 138-139
        dips, 139-140
        lateral pull downs, 135, 137
        leg curls, 145-146
        leg extensions, 147-148
        leg presses, 134-135
        lower-body workouts, 145
        seated biceps curls, 142
        shoulder presses, 141
        triceps push downs, 143
        upper-body workouts, 133-134
        upright rows, 137
    45-minute cardiovascular, 163
        bike riding, 162
        cross-country ski machines, 164-165
        elliptical trainers, 163-164
        rowing machines, 162-163
        running, 159-162
    45-minute strength-training
        abductors, 175
        adductors, 176
        concentration curls, 186
        decline presses, 180-181
        dumbbell rows, 183-184
        flyes, 168-169
        incline presses, 179
        lateral raises, 170-171
        lower-body workouts, 172-173
        oblique crunches, 171
        shrugs, 185
        split routines, 178-179, 183
        squats, 173-174
        standing calf raises, 177

triceps kickbacks, 182
upper-body workouts,
  167-168
45-minute total body, 152
  cardiovascular, 154-155
  cool downs, 155-156
  strength training, 157
  stretching, 156-157
  warm-ups, 152-154
60-minute cardiovascular
  bike riding, 201-203
  classes, 204-205
  having fun, 206
  running, 198-201
60-minute strength-training
  full-body workouts, 208
  lower-body emphasis
    routines, 211-212
  push/pull split routines,
    212-218
  seated calf raises, 208-209
  upper-body emphasis
    routines, 209-211
60-minute total body, 190
  cardiovascular, 190-193
  strength training, 193-194
  stretching, 194
after work, 20-21
bad weather, 258-259
benefits, 7
cardiovascular exercise
  cross-training, 236-237
  health, 22-23
  pitfalls, 222-223
cautions
  asthma, 30-31
  diabetes, 29-30
  hypertension, 29
cycling, 238-239
daily routines, 16-18
detraining, 40
developing habits, 9
endorphins, 10
equipment, 71-73
excuses for not working out, 14
exercise classes, 62
expectations, 4-5
fartlek, 127
feeling sluggish, 9-10
full-body, routines, 70-71
goals, 22
golf, 241-242
habits, 9
health benefits, 7-11
high altitudes, 257-258
hydration, 61
key points, 5-7
length of workout, 4-5
lifting, speed of movement, 70

lunchtime routines, 20
martial arts, 245-246
meals, 61
missing workouts, 14
morning routines, 18-19
mothers, 95-96
obstacles, time investments,
  5-7
office
  calisthenics, 272-273
  contract/relax techniques,
    273
  stairs, 271-272
  strength training, 270-271
  stretching, 267-269
overtraining, 40
paddling, 246-247
partners, 94
physical benefits, 11
physical health, 95-96
psychological benefits, 10-11
quizzes, 5-7
repititions, 70
routines, 70-71
schmoozing, 4-5
seasonal
  summer, 290-295
  winter, 288-290
sets and reps, 70
setting goals, 22
short workouts, 5-7
skating, 242-243
skiing, 244-245
snowboarding, 244-245
socializing, 4-5
something vs. nothing, 5-7
specific fitness goals, 22
strength training, 69-71
  crunches, 226
  pitfalls, 225-233
stress management, 7-9
stretching pitfalls, 223-225
tennis, 239, 241
terminology, gymspeak, 70
therapeutic benefits, 7-8
time management, 14-18
traveling, 21-22, 252-254
  calisthenics, 253
  chin-ups, 254
  jumping rope, 253
  pull-ups, 254
  push-ups, 253-254
  resistance bands, 254
treadmill, 127
values-based prioritizing,
  24-25
work out at work, 21
workstations, posture, 265-266

yoga
  dress codes, 281
  plough, pitfalls, 225
  stretching, 87
yogurt, 50

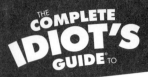
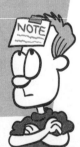